1996

D1033813

High-Performance Nutrition

Other Books by the Authors

Books coauthored by Susan M. Kleiner, Ph.D., R.D.:

The High Performance Cookbook
The High Performance Vegetarian Cookbook

Books coauthored by Maggie Greenwood-Robinson:

BUILT! The New Bodybuilding for Everyone
Lean Bodies
Lean Bodies Total Fitness
High-Performance Bodybuilding
John Parrillo's 50 Workout Secrets
Shape Training

High-Performance Nutrition

The Total Eating Plan to Maximize Your Workout

Susan M. Kleiner, Ph.D., R.D.
Maggie Greenwood-Robinson

John Wiley & Sons, Inc.
New York • Chichester • Brisbane • Toronto • Singapore

This text is printed on acid-free paper.

Copyright © 1996 by Susan M. Kleiner and Maggie Greenwood-Robinson
Personal diet and training logs copyright © 1996 by Susan M. Kleiner

Published by John Wiley & Sons, Inc.

All rights reserved. Published simultaneously in Canada.

Reproduction or translation of any part of this work beyond that permitted by Section 107 or 108 of the 1976 United States Copyright Act without the permission of the copyright owner is unlawful. Requests for permission or further information should be addressed to the Permissions Department, John Wiley & Sons, Inc.

The information contained in this book is not intended to serve as a replacement for the advice of a physician. Any use of the information set forth in this book is at the reader's discretion. The author and publisher specifically disclaim any and all liability arising directly from the use or application of any information contained in this book. A health care professional should be consulted prior to following any new diet.

The authors would like to thank the following athletes, all of whom agreed to be featured in case histories for this book: Al "Bubba" Baker, Joanne Bowser, Stephen Douglass, Gail Friedberg, Matt Lawrence, Todd Martin, and Marla Ridenour.

The "Determine" checklist (page 208) is reprinted with permission by the Nutrition Screening Initiative, a project of the American Academy of Family Physicians, the American Dietetic Association, and the National Council on Aging, Inc., and funded in part by a grant from Ross Products Division, Abbott Laboratories.

ISBN 0-471-11520-7

Printed in the United States of America
10   9   8   7   6   5   4   3   2   1

To Mom and Dad: You gave me my inner strength.

Contents

Acknowledgments

High-Performance Nutrition: The Total Eating Plan to Maximize Your Workout has become a reality rather than a personal dream due to the combined efforts of some remarkably visionary individuals.

To Maggie Greenwood-Robinson—thank you for an extraordinary collaboration that has been both a joy and a success. I look forward to many more.

To Madeleine Morel, our agent—your direction and support have been invaluable.

To PJ Dempsey, our editor at John Wiley & Sons—thank you for the opportunity to put what I practice into print.

Finally, to my family—thank you for your love and tolerance through my years of preparing for this book. Without you, it would still be a dream.

—S.M.K.

Preface

I became interested in sports nutrition for one simple reason: As someone who's athletic, with an ever-active lifestyle, I need the staying power to work—and to work out. As I pursued my career in sports nutrition, I found it frustrating to be able to find so much information about what to eat for endurance sports or exercise, but so little for a person like me who strength-trains or cross-trains with a variety of different activities. And so I made it my personal quest to create a nutrition program that would fit all types of exercisers—strength trainers, cross trainers, aerobic exercisers, and recreational athletes. This book is the culmination of what I have learned through working with all types of athletes, conducting my own research, and sifting through the credible research of other top sports scientists.

The turning point in my understanding of exercise and health came after I began working with drug-free bodybuilders and football players. If you're neither, you're probably wondering what you have in common with them. Please read on.

Working with drug-free bodybuilders was a real eye-opener. When I began researching bodybuilders in 1982, only a handful of scientific articles had been written about strength trainers. The few existing articles zeroed in on how unhealthy bodybuilders were because of their abuse of anabolic steroids, which are tissue-building drugs. Through my research, I recognized that not only were bodybuilders incredible athletes, but those who trained without drugs were very healthy despite a relatively high fat diet. In those days, bodybuilders did not include aerobic exercise in their regular training routines, and they were unaware of the sources of hidden fat in the diet. Despite this, they were very heart healthy, with good aerobic capacity, cholesterol profiles, and blood pressure levels. And they were very lean. The common denominator in their good health was their mode of exercise—strength training. I became convinced that strength-training exercise is as important to maintaining health as aerobic exercise has proven to be. Not just for bodybuilders, but for everyone.

Football players have nearly the same dietary problems as most Americans do. They lead busy lives. They're on the road. They don't have control over all their meals. They might skip a meal. And they eat too much fat. Because they are highly active, they can handle the calories without gaining as much weight on a high-fat diet as most people would. All athletes, however, perform better on a high-carbohydrate diet. And so will you.

Retired football players are notorious for continuing to indulge in high-fat diets. The problem is, they are no longer active enough to handle those extra fat calories. Now they're in the same boat as a lot of Americans: a sedentary life with a fatty diet. This lifestyle usually leads to obesity and high risks for chronic diseases. I was able to successfully get most of the players I worked with to modify their diets with very little pain at all. I did this by making simple, low-fat changes in certain recipes and focusing on what they could eat, not what they couldn't. I gave them tips on how to shop, cook, and eat on the road. These techniques worked out so well with football players that I began using them with other clients and achieving the same degree of success.

With *High-Performance Nutrition*, I've been able to codify what I've learned in the past fifteen years of working with athletes and exercisers into a program that will give you energy and endurance, plus provide the nutrients your body needs to get in shape and stay healthy. This nutrition book provides valid, comprehensive information on how diet and nutrition affect fat loss, muscular development, strength increases, workout stamina, and disease prevention for those engaged in a regular exercise program or competitive sports. It truly is the total nutrition plan for today's active person.

—Susan M. Kleiner, Ph.D., R.D.

How to Use This Book

This book is a nutrition guide for physically active people of all ages—exercisers, strength trainers, cross trainers, recreational athletes, and endurance athletes. Nutrition for the physically active person has two critical components: nutrition for performance and nutrition for long-term health. I really must underscore the latter, especially when you consider that five of the leading causes of death in the United States—heart disease, stroke, cancer, diabetes, and digestive disorders—are all linked to poor nutrition. You certainly can't be physically active if you're stricken with a life-shortening illness. The same nutrition that gives you the energy and endurance for exercise, training, and competition keeps you going strong on the health front as well.

I have organized the book around seven main parts, including what high-performance living means, foods for physically active people, supplementation for physically active people, controversial supplements, fluid needs of exercisers and athletes, weight control, and nutrition for special needs (vegetarians, pregnant women, and aging adults). Under each part are chapters that cover specific nutritional subjects of relevance to exercisers and athletes. Part One, for example, discusses the benefits of aerobics, strength training, and cross training, plus several of the key nutritional issues that apply to each. Part Two contains chapters that cover the nutrients in our foods and how they enhance performance and promote long-term health.

Specific information pertinent to your workout and training needs is easy to find. If you're interested in supplements, for example, look through Part Three, where you'll find chapters on antioxidant supplements, a breakthrough supplement known as creatine, and my special firming formula, which creates an environment conducive to muscle toning and development following your workout. Other chapters within the book discuss unproven supplements, herbal supplements, caffeine, water, sports drinks, fat-loss strategies, artificial sweeteners and fat replacers, the role of exercise in fat loss, lifestyle diet planning, gaining weight, vegetarian nutrition, nutrition for pregnancy, and nutritional issues of interest to specific age groups.

My Thirty-Day High-Performance Menu Plan is found in appendix A. It contains 1,800-calorie and 3,000-calorie plans, along with easy-to-prepare recipes. The plan tells you exactly what to eat each day of the week. You don't have to worry about the nutrition, either. All the nutrients you need for vitality and good health are built right into the plan. You can adapt these menus to match the nutritional requirements of your sport or exercise choice, too. Along with the plan, you'll find the top seventy foods you need to achieve peak performance.

Appendix B features my High-Performance Nutrition Prescription Chart in which you can find—at a glance—exactly how to eat, drink, and supplement for endurance exercise, strength training, and cross training. This chart capsulizes the key nutritional principles relevant to active people in a convenient, easy-to-follow format.

Other appendixes include information for special circumstances, such as how to eat while you're on the mend from a sports injury: how to properly take medications, food, and nutritional supplements; how to plan your daily diet and training schedule; and, finally, how to make wiser, healthier purchases of food based on its additive content.

Much of the nutritional information in this book is cutting edge, thanks to an ever-expanding base of research on nutrition for cross trainers and strength trainers. I've balanced that research with real-life stories from my own practice that show how exercisers, professional athletes, Olympic contenders, and corporate CEOs are successfully applying my diet strategies. Armed with this just-discovered yet practical information, you'll learn how to maintain high performance for the rest of your life.

PART ONE

WHAT HIGH-PERFORMANCE LIVING MEANS

CHAPTER 1

Eating for Performance and Health

The New Nutrition for Physically Active People

Are you "going strong"? I mean, do you feel energetic, productive, and healthy? Do you perform well in your sport, or are you trailing the pack? Is your body trim and toned, or has it turned to pure pudge?

If you feel healthy and in great shape, congratulations. You *are* going strong. But if you're like most people, there's probably some room for improvement.

It's safe to say that everyone, regardless of age, wants to enjoy high-performance living—have energy and endurance for exercise, competition, work, and play, and be healthy and resist disease. High-performance living means staying vibrant, healthy, and in shape at every stage of your life.

How, then, do you maintain high performance? In two ways—by staying active and eating right. Sounds simple enough, but the problem is that most active people have their nutrition all wrong. They're not following the right diet for their exercise or sport, or they're resorting to gimmicky diets to get in shape. It's practically impossible to reach your fitness goals without the proper nutrition program to get you there.

Today people are working out and training much differently. Until recently, exercise meant a jog in the park, a few laps around the neighborhood, or some weekly aerobics classes to tune up the heart. Now such measures aren't enough for total fitness. More of us are now "cross-training," with a combination of workouts: cardiovascular training for heart health, strength training to tone muscles, and recreational sports like hiking for the pure fun of it. Even athletes like runners and marathoners cross-train for a particular competitive event by lifting weights to get stronger for their sport.

The Rewards of High-Performance Nutrition

The rules of the exercise game have clearly changed. But so have the rules for nutrition. The one-diet-fits-all approach to nutrition for exercise and sports no longer applies. There are specific ways to eat and supplement for your exercise and training routine. If you cross-train, for example, you may benefit from increasing the amount of protein and carbohydrate you eat. Or if you're an endurance athlete, your performance will improve considerably by following the carbohydrate-loading method described in chapter 3. And if you strength-train, use my nutritional tricks to maximize your energy reserves during workouts—and give your body the nutrients it needs to develop lean muscle. By matching the right dietary principle to your activity, you can do the following:

- Train longer and harder
- Delay fatigue
- Help your body recover faster after working out
- Perform much better overall
- Guard your health against life-threatening illnesses
- Reverse some of the physical signs of aging

All these rewards are precisely what high-performance living is all about.

The Benefits of Exercise

Perhaps right now you're a "one-exercise" person, or maybe you've already recognized the fitness rewards of doing two or more types of exercise. Whatever the case, let's take a closer look at the benefits derived from aerobic exercise, strength training, and cross training, plus some of the nutritional principles that apply to each one.

Aerobic and Endurance Exercise

Aerobic exercise is the kind that gets your heart pumping. Examples include walking, jogging, running, swimming, bicycling, and aerobic dancing. This kind of exercise has enormous benefits. For example:

- A boost in aerobic capacity—the amount of oxygen you use during a minute of exercise. Aerobic exercise produces positive changes in the heart and circulation. As a result, your body can better transport oxygen-carrying blood to working muscles.
- Reduced risk of dying from heart disease.
- An increase in the blood level of high-density lipoprotein (HDL) cholesterol—the type that protects your heart from disease.
- Protection against osteoporosis by building bone mass.
- Stronger immune function and better resistance to disease. Aerobic exercise stimulates the immune system by producing antibodies and virus-fighting cells.

- Fat burning. Aerobic exercise speeds the transfer of oxygen from the blood into the muscles. This increase in blood flow helps muscles burn fat more efficiently. Aerobic exercise also increases the activity of fat-burning enzymes.

Nutrition for Aerobic Exercisers and Endurance Athletes

Aerobic and endurance exercise is "sustained" activity, meaning that you continue it for many minutes at a time without rest. This type of energy demand relies on adequate body stores of fat and carbohydrate, plus sufficient vitamins and minerals to regulate the release of energy. If you're training for competition, you may need additional calories to fuel your body during periods of greater energy expenditure. Intense training also breaks down body tissues; therefore, you need to know what to eat—and when to eat it—to repair this breakdown and initiate recovery. By selecting foods and supplements wisely, you can get all the nutrients you need to fuel your body, build it up, and stimulate the energy systems used during aerobic exercise. You'll learn how to do that by following the nutritional principles outlined in this book.

Most of the available information on nutrition for active people is intended for endurance athletes and aerobic exercisers. If you fit in this category, you probably know that certain foods, particularly carbohydrates, maximize performance. Nonetheless, it has been my experience that even the most elite endurance athletes have misconceptions about what to eat. In other words, there's still more for you to learn about aerobic nutrition!

Let me give you an example: Todd M., a twenty-three-year-old runner, was preparing to compete in the 1996 Olympic marathon trials. For his level of training, he had a poorly planned diet: water only before his morning run, some lunch around 10:15 A.M., no food before his afternoon workout, dinner at 5:30 P.M., and occasionally a snack before bedtime. His average dietary intake was 4,700 calories, with 16 percent of those calories coming from protein, 59 percent from carbohydrates, and 25 percent from fat.

Todd had been gaining some body fat and was concerned about it. Here was a case in which an athlete was eating too many calories—about five hundred more a day than he really needed. Far too many of those calories were from fat. As you'll find out later, the type of calories you eat makes a big difference in weight control. To offset the calorie surplus, I suggested that Todd start lifting weights. This type of exercise, referred to as "strength training," would also add some muscle to his frame, giving him more strength and power for his sport.

Another major nutritional booby trap in his diet was not fueling himself properly before and after both training and competition. I overhauled his diet to correct this problem. Following my recommendations, Todd upped his intake of carbohydrates to 65 percent of his total daily calories. He began fueling himself before training and races with high-carbohydrate snacks and sports drinks. During events lasting an hour or more, he'd drink at least 4 oz. of a fluid replacement beverage every fifteen to twenty minutes. Within two hours after each race, Todd drank a high-carbohydrate supplement to restock his muscles with energy-giving glycogen.

After sticking to this program, Todd reported back to me within a year that he had made major gains in speed, energy, and overall performance.

Like Todd, maybe you compete in an endurance sport or do aerobic exercise on a regular basis, but you're puzzled by your lackluster performance and low energy levels. Chances are it's a nutritional problem—like not eating enough carbohydrates at critical times. I work with endurance athletes and exercisers all the time who are committed to training and working out, but they just don't fuel themselves properly. As Todd learned, you can attain high performance in your sport by making a few key adjustments in your nutrition.

Strength Training

Strength training is any kind of weight-bearing activity in which your muscles are challenged to work harder each time they're exercised. Examples of strength training include lifting weights, working out on weight-training machines, performing calisthenics, and exercising with special rubber bands.

With strength training, you're developing and preserving muscle, a vital body tissue. Working together, muscles move the 206 bones in your body. About 42 percent of your body weight is muscle if you're a man; 36 percent if you're a woman. The energy for movement is produced inside muscle cells, where nutrients are chemically converted into fuel. In strength training, two types of energy systems are called into play. High-energy phosphates (compounds inside muscle cells) are used in the first few moments of muscle contractions, and muscle glycogen, which is stored carbohydrate, is used in short bouts of exercise lasting one to three minutes.

Strength training is to the nineties what aerobic exercise was to the eighties. The reason is that strength training carries with it many newly discovered benefits that are just now coming to light. We've known for decades that this form of exercise strengthens muscles for improved athletic performance. But its benefits go far beyond athletics. We now know this amazing fact: Our bodies need strong muscles for lifelong health.

Myoatrophy   Between the ages of twenty and seventy, you can lose about 20 percent of your muscle—a condition technically known as *myoatrophy* (my-o-AT-ro-fee). Myoatrophy is more dramatic in men, but women begin to lose significant amounts of muscle after menopause. The health consequences of myoatrophy are serious, even life-threatening. As long as you stay physically active, eat right, and include strength training in your workout, you prevent myoatrophy. This has tremendous payoffs both now and in the future. Let's look at some of the benefits of keeping in excellent muscular shape with strength training and proper nutrition.

Staying Lean and Fit

Muscle is the active tissue in your body. The more muscle you have, the faster your metabolic rate, the speed at which chemical reactions like calorie burning and respiration take place. If you don't have much muscle, your metabolism runs in low gear. Fewer calories are burned, and fat pounds can pile on.

Too much body fat paves the way to obesity. Obesity is a risk factor for heart disease, diabetes, high blood pressure, certain cancers, digestive illnesses, and other life-shortening diseases. By strength training and following the nutritional guidelines in this book, you'll stay lean, muscularly fit, and prevent unwanted pounds from piling on.

Preventing Diabetes

Diabetes is a sugar metabolism disorder in which there's a glut of glucose (blood sugar) in the blood. Though treatable, diabetes has health-threatening complications, including stroke, heart attack, kidney disease, gangrene of the feet, blindness, and nerve damage. It's the seventh leading cause of death in the United States, and about 11 million people have it.

Under normal circumstances, glucose circulates in the blood and is transported to muscle cells, fat cells, and other cells where it can be used for fuel. To enter the cells, glucose needs help from insulin, a hormone produced in the pancreas. Once insulin gets to the outer surface of the cell, it acts like a key and unlocks tiny receptors surrounding the cell. The cell opens up and lets glucose in for use as food.

Sometimes normal insulin activity is upset, and cells can't use glucose properly. Either not enough insulin is produced (a condition known as Type I diabetes) or the cells aren't letting in enough glucose for proper nourishment (Type II diabetes). Type I diabetics require injections of insulin.

With age, your body gradually loses its ability to regulate glucose. This puts you in danger of developing Type II diabetes, which can typically occur in people over forty years old, particularly among those who are overweight. In fact, more than 80 percent of Type II diabetics are overweight. What's more, Type II diabetes is present in 25 percent of the population age eighty-five and older. Sufferers have normal concentrations of insulin, but their bodies don't handle it well.

Exercise may help you steer clear of Type II diabetes as you get older and control it if you already have it. Muscle cells are sensitive to insulin. Maintaining muscle tissue helps normalize the flow of glucose from the blood into muscle cells where it can be properly used for energy. We don't know exactly what happens at the cellular level, but somehow more glucose is able to get inside cells if you exercise regularly and develop your muscles.

Preventing Osteoporosis

No doubt you've heard of osteoporosis. This bone-thinning disease is a debilitating, sometimes fatal disorder in which vital mincrals like calcium leach from your bones as you age. The good news is that weight-bearing exercise strengthens the skeleton by stimulating the bone to produce new cells.

Where does myoatrophy fit into the picture? Among the main constituents of muscle tissue are nitrogen and the mineral potassium. As much as 60 percent of the body's potassium is found in your muscles, and there's more nitrogen in muscles than in any other tissue. Scientists can tell how much muscle is lost with age by measuring losses of nitrogen and potassium from the muscle.

Recent studies have found that age-related losses of body nitrogen are closely linked to losses in body calcium. This finding suggests that if you're losing muscle as you age, vital calcium is exiting your bones, too, and osteoporosis could result.

The point I want to emphasize is that muscle loss precedes bone loss. All the attention focused on osteoporosis has raised a much-needed awareness about this crippling disease—and communicated ways to fight it. That's good. But we've really put the cart before the horse on this health issue. Myoatrophy needs to be reckoned with initially. By preserving your muscle, you take the first—and very critical—step toward preventing bone loss.

Clearly, myoatrophy is a very serious medical problem. Yet it doesn't get serious attention. It should be emphasized and publicized as a leading disorder of aging, just as osteoporosis has been. Americans then need to learn what can be done to prevent it—and ultimately all the other diseases it produces.

Dispelling the Myths

Despite all the benefits of strength training, a lot of people are hesitant to try strength training. They're deterred by certain myths surrounding it. Let me dispel some of those right now.

Myth #1   Strength training will build big, bulky muscles.   This is the number one fear among women. They're scared to death of building bulky muscles, so they shy away from strength training altogether. If you're a woman who starts strength training, your body composition will change. You'll become more toned and better defined, with less body fat. But rest assured: You won't bulk up like men do. The reason is hormones; your body doesn't make enough male hormones to produce large muscles.

Myth #2   Strength training makes you gain weight.   True, but it's muscle weight, and that's what you want. Lean, toned, tight muscle. Pound for pound, muscle weighs twice as much as fat. That's why weighing yourself on a scale doesn't give an accurate reading of lean tissue gained or fat pounds lost. Opt instead for some form of body composition testing. See chapter 17 for information on how to check your body fat percentage.

In reality, strength training keeps you trim. With a regular strength-training program, 85 percent of every pound you lose while watching your weight is pure fat. Your body gets firmer and leaner as a result of consistently working out.

Myth #3   If you stop strength training, muscle turns to fat.   Muscle and fat are two different types of tissue. Neither can magically transform into the other. The reason you plump up after stopping strength training is a shift in body composition. Muscle shrinks, and energy needs decrease accordingly. Most people don't adjust their calories to meet the reduced energy needs, so body fat starts creeping back on.

Strength-Training Nutrition

The goals of strength training are to get stronger, develop lean muscle, and prevent myoatrophy. To achieve those goals, you have to take in adequate calories, carbohydrates, protein, vitamins, and minerals. It takes about 2,500 calories to form a pound of muscle, and the additional calories to do that should come primarily from carbohydrates like grains, breads, fruits, and vegetables. It may come as a surprise to you that I emphasize carbs, since these are associated more with endurance exercise than with strength training. In fact, when most people think of strength training, they immediately think of protein.

But carbs are key. The intensity of most strength-training routines can rapidly use up most of the carbohydrate stored in the muscles, leading to fatigue. When this happens, endurance and performance suffer. Muscle can't be developed without the fuel to drive activity. By upping carbohydrates to levels as high or higher than endurance athletes typically eat, a strength trainer can outperform even the strongest person in the gym.

Protein is still an important nutritional issue in strength training, however, since this nutrient is directly involved in building body tissues. New discoveries in the science of sports nutrition have finally cleared the air on how much protein strength trainers really need, and there are very specific protein requirements. If you don't eat enough protein, your body can't make new muscle or adequately repair the tissue that breaks down with training.

The entire research base on nutrition for strength trainers has greatly expanded. In addition to carbohydrate and protein issues, we now know more than ever about how the right nutrient mix—supplements included—can support the muscle-development process and build the energy systems of your body. If your nutrition is subpar on calories and nutrients, you'll see minimal results at best, and you may actually lose lean muscle. But by following the nutritional guidelines for strength trainers explained in this book, you'll make remarkable progress in how you look and feel. Plus you'll help protect yourself from myoatrophy-related health problems later in life.

Cross Training

Cross training involves doing a combination of activities—for example, adding two strength-training workouts to your four-day-a-week running program or playing tennis twice a week, along with some aerobic dance classes. Cross training gives you plenty of variety in your fitness program and ensures that all muscle groups, plus your cardiovascular system, get a full workout. Endurance athletes know that strength training makes them better runners, marathoners, triathletes, rowers, or swimmers. Likewise, strength athletes know that aerobic training builds their oxygen-delivery system, helps keep body fat to a minimum, and improves overall cardiovascular health. Without question, cross training combines the best of both strength training and aerobic training. The benefits of all these fitness programs are summarized for you in table 1-1. If you want to cross-train but haven't added an aerobics or strength-training component to your fitness program yet, see chapter 21 for information on how to start either type of exercise.

Table 1-1

HEALTH BENEFITS OF EXERCISE

Strength Training	Aerobics
Less body fat	Less body fat
More lean muscle	Faster metabolism
Faster metabolism	Better weight control and management
Better weight control and management	Improved capacity to use oxygen
Prevention of age-related myoatrophy	Greater endurance
Greater bone strength and density	Improved flexibility
Prevention of osteoporosis	Prevention of osteoporosis
Greater muscle strength	Improved cardiovascular function
Greater muscular endurance	Protection against coronary heart disease
Improved flexibility	Improved cholesterol profiles
Delayed aging	Slower heart rate
Improved cardiovascular function	Lower blood pressure
Improved cholesterol profiles	Better coordination and balance
Increased mobility	Improved blood sugar regulation
Improved blood sugar regulation	Strengthened immune system
Improved body image	Less depression and anxiety
Extension of active lifetime	Extension of active lifetime

Cross Training

Cross training provides all of the above benefits, plus improved sports performance and the variety to keep your exercise motivation high.

Cross-Training Nutrition

When you do a combination of activities, many nutritional issues come into play. One of the most critical is calories. If you're an athlete who has recently added strength training to your training, you have to pay even greater attention to the number of calories you're eating daily. The extra energy expended means you need more calories to fuel your workouts. If you don't eat the required calories every day, and in the right proportions, then you're running in low gear. You could lose weight, become ill, injure yourself, or suffer a loss in performance. Preventing such complications is as easy as fueling yourself with enough calories from the right nutrients.

Many people cross-train purely to improve their physical fitness, and the goal of weight management often tops their fitness wish list. They know that nutrition is critical to weight control and appearance, yet they still plan their diets based on myths and misconceptions, trying fad diets, unproven supplements, and the like.

Football players, who are cross-training athletes in the truest sense of the word, are a good example. Several years ago I worked as the nutritionist for the Cleveland Browns. My experience with this NFL team illustrates some common problems relating to nutrition and weight control.

Football players are constantly waging the body weight war. Depending on the coach, players may be asked to gain weight any way they can, gain only muscle, lose weight slowly, or shed some pounds by next week. As team nutritionist, my job was to help the players shape up—and do it in a healthy manner. This wasn't always so easy. Like overzealous dieters, some players starved and dehydrated themselves to make weight. Others gorged themselves with the wrong foods to gain weight. Not only are these practices unhealthy, they also set up athletes for injuries during practice or play.

With my program, you'll learn a very different approach to weight management—one that builds health rather than tears it down. You don't have to sacrifice good nutrition, either, since very few foods are excluded from the diet. If you want to eat dessert, drink a glass of wine, splurge occasionally, fine. I build your indulgences and favorite foods into a diet plan tailored just for you. Sure, there are some things that are off-limits on a daily basis. In other words, you can eat anything you want once in a while, but not every day.

You'll learn what I've been teaching my clients for years: how to create your own high-performance diet and prepare delicious low-fat recipes to go along with it. This approach works—the weight stays off, performance remains intact, and you head off potential health risks at the pass.

Nutrition and Long-term Health

If you're successful in using the diet and nutrition principles in this book, you'll stay healthier, develop lean, healthy muscle, heal more readily after injuries, maintain a higher level of performance year after year, and possibly extend your athletic and your active lifetime.

But there's another payoff: long-term health. As someone who is active, your sole concern today may be your appearance or your physical performance. But perhaps you're also concerned about how healthy you'll be in the future. I'm sure you want to be as active ten or twenty years from now as you are today. That's where nutrition plays a part.

Without good nutrition, you're setting yourself up for health problems later on. As mentioned earlier, five of the ten leading causes of death in the United States—heart disease, stroke, cancer, diabetes, and digestive disorders—are linked to poor nutrition.

You don't have to be a victim of vitality-robbing illnesses—as long as you take the right steps now. I'll let you in on a little secret: Aging is mostly an accumulation of bad eating habits and inactivity over a lifetime. According to the Canada Health Survey, leading a sedentary life now means about ten years of partial dependency later and a final year of total dependency as your life nears its end. That's certainly nothing to look forward to.

Some good news: You can delay, even avoid, many of the pitfalls of aging by taking care of yourself throughout your life. The foods you eat and the exercise you do both play a part in keeping you active and healthy—for a lifetime.

PART TWO

FOODS FOR PHYSICALLY ACTIVE PEOPLE

CHAPTER 2

Carbohydrates

The Energy Food

You put gas in your car, keep it well lubricated with oil, and periodically check the levels of transmission, brake, and other fluids so that things keep running longer and better. But do you give the same consideration to the vital fuels that power your body?

Among the fuels your body runs on are carbohydrates, organic compounds that contain carbon, hydrogen, and oxygen atoms in various combinations. Carbs are to your body what gas is to a car—the fuel that gets you going. In fact, the major role of carbohydrates in nutrition is to provide energy. During exercise, carbohydrates are one of your main sources of energy.

How Carbohydrates Work

Carbohydrates can be thought of as molecular necklaces with the carbon, oxygen, and hydrogen atoms strung together in chains. These necklaces are broken apart during digestion by digestive enzymes and converted into individual beads or molecules of blood glucose, also known as blood sugar. Assisted by the hormone insulin, blood glucose is ushered into cells to be used by various tissues in the body.

Several things can happen to glucose. Once inside a cell, it can be quickly metabolized to supply energy, particularly for the brain and other parts of the nervous system that depend on glucose for fuel. Or it may be converted to either liver or muscle glycogen, the storage form of carbohydrate. When you exercise or use your muscles, the body mobilizes muscle glycogen for energy. Blood glucose can also turn into body fat and get packed away in fat tissue. This happens when you eat more carbohydrates than you need or than your body can store as liver or muscle glycogen.

Types of Carbohydrates

There are two types of carbs—complex carbohydrates and simple carbohydrates—and each plays a different role in your health.

1. *Complex carbohydrates,* also called starches, are created when three or more glucose molecules combine. Most plant foods, including cereals, pasta, fruits, and vegetables, are complex carbohydrates. They're packed with nutrients, including dietary fiber, an indigestible carbohydrate that has a long list of impressive health benefits.

2. *Simple carbohydrates,* otherwise known as sugars, are subdivided into two categories: monosaccharides and disaccharides. The three major monosaccharides are glucose, fructose, and galactose. Glucose and fructose are found mostly in fruits, and galactose is found in milk.

   When two monosaccharides link up chemically, a disaccharide is formed. A pairing of galactose and glucose, for example, yields the milk sugar lactose. Ordinary table sugar is a disaccharide called sucrose.

Is Sugar Harmful?

Sugar, or sucrose, is a major source of calories but a highly refined food that offers no nutrients to go along with the calories. For this reason, nutritionists describe sugar as having "empty calories." Because sugar contains no nutrients other than calories, it's best to limit it in your diet. Too much sugar has been associated with tooth decay, obesity, cardiovascular disease, and blood sugar metabolism disorders such as diabetes and hypoglycemia.

Should Athletes Eat Sugar?

Some people mistakenly believe that eating simple sugars just prior to an athletic event provides instant energy and therefore improves performance. Quite the contrary. First, concentrated sugar in the stomach can actually hold fluid in the stomach, and this creates an uncomfortable feeling. Second, sugar can cause a fast hike in blood sugar levels, followed by a fast drop, leaving you sluggish and fatigued. This hike in blood sugar stimulates the secretion of insulin, which accelerates the body's use of muscle glycogen. If your glycogen levels are depleted too early in a race, you'll barely make it to the finish line. Clearly, no case can be made for eating simple sugars prior to training or competing.

Hidden Sugar

As for the rest of your diet, you may be eating more sugar than you think, even if a food is labeled *No Sugar Added.* Legally, the only ingredient that must be called sugar on a label is sucrose. A food could still contain simple sugars like honey, molasses, corn syrup, or fructose. By law, none of these are required to be labeled as sugar.

Table 2-1 describes many of the different forms of sugars found in food. Even more sugars, such as sorbitol, xylitol, and mannitol, are added to foods, but they are known more generally as non-cavity-promoting, low-calorie sweeteners. (For more information on low-calorie and artificial sweeteners, see chapter 20.)

Be a wise consumer. The next time you see *No Sugar Added* on a food label, read the fine print. Make sure that you know what you're buying, and what you're eating.

Table 2-1

SIMPLE SUGARS FOUND IN PROCESSED FOODS

Sugar (sucrose)	Refined crystallized sap of the sugar cane or sugar beet; a combination of glucose and fructose; less sweet than fructose.
Dextrose (glucose)	A simple sugar made of only one molecule; less sweet than fructose or sucrose.
Lactose	A simple sugar from milk; less sweet than sucrose, fructose, or maltose.
Maltose	A simple sugar made from starch; less sweet than sucrose or fructose.
Maltodextrin	A manufactured sugar from maltose and dextrose.
Brown sugar	A refined sugar coated with molasses. The minerals calcium, iron, and potassium are present in this sugar.
Raw sugar	A less refined sugar that still has some natural molasses coating.
Fructose	A simple sugar refined from fruit; the sweetest sugar of all.
Molasses	The syrup separated from sugar crystals during the refining process. Blackstrap molasses is a good source of calcium, iron, and potassium.
Honey	A concentrated solution of fructose and glucose (80%) and some sucrose.
Maple syrup	A concentrated sap from sugar maple trees, predominantly fructose.
Corn syrup	A manufactured syrup of corn starch, containing varying proportions of glucose, maltose, and dextrose.
High-fructose corn syrup	A highly concentrated syrup of predominantly fructose.
White grape juice	A highly purified fructose solution; virtually no other nutrients are present.

Clearing Up the Confusion over Carbohydrates

In 1995 the results of multiple hospital and university studies turned the carbo-hydrate story on its ear. The findings suggested that some people (about 25 per-cent of the population) are "carbohydrate sensitive"—a condition in which calo-ries from certain kinds of starchy carbohydrates, particularly the more processed types like pasta and bread, are easily converted to stored body fat. After a carbo-hydrate meal, the body overproduces insulin, stimulating the liver to turn glucose into fat.

Should you be concerned about eating pasta and bread? No! This bodily re-sponse does not affect 75 percent of the population, and the effect is primarily lim-ited to very overweight people, who tend to have blood sugar problems anyway. If you think you have a blood sugar problem, consult your physician, who should be able to diagnose it and prescribe the proper treatment.

In any event, you should be eating a variety of complex carbs like beans and whole grains, in addition to breads and pasta. Even if you're carbohydrate sensi-tive, the variety minimizes the effects. Also, staying active helps control body weight—and builds muscle tissue, which helps normalize the body's use of glu-cose.

Carbohydrate Requirements

Ideally, for most physically active people, 60 to 65 percent of the calories in their diet should come from carbohydrates, particularly complex carbs. Strength train-ers may need a little more, as I explain in the next chapter. The best way to in-crease complex carbohydrates is to add foods like whole grain cereals and breads, pasta, rice, potatoes, yams, legumes and other vegetables and fruits to your diet.

Here's how to determine your carbohydrate needs, assuming a 2,000-calorie diet:

Step 1: Multiply your total daily calories by 65 percent (.65). For example: 2,000 calories × .65 = 1,300.

Step 2: Divide your daily carb calories by 4, the number of grams in each gram of carbohydrate. Returning to the example: 1,300 ÷ 4 = 425 g total car-bohydrate for the day.

Another way to determine your personal carb needs is by eating 3 to 5 g of carbohydrate for every pound of your body weight. But if counting grams sounds like too much of a hassle, just design your diet based on eating high-carb foods most of the time. You'll have just enough room left over for the protein you need and a minimal amount of fat.

Table 2-2, which provides the number of grams found in servings of healthy food sources of carbohydrates, will help you track and figure out the correct amount of carbs to include in your daily diet. Also see my Thirty-Day High-Performance Menu Plan in Appendix A. It provides an 1,800-calorie diet and a 3,000-calorie diet in which 65 percent of the calories come from carbohydrates.

Table 2-2

GOOD FOOD SOURCES OF CARBOHYDRATES

Food	Amount	Carbohydrates (grams)
Fruits		
Apple	1 medium	21
Orange	1 medium	15
Banana	1 medium	27
Raisins	¼ cup	29
Apricots, dried	10 halves	22
Fruit Roll-Up	2	24
Vegetables		
Corn, canned	½ cup	18
Winter squash	½ cup	15
Tomato sauce, Ragú	½ cup	10
Peas	½ cup	10
Carrot	1 medium	7
Bread-Type Foods		
Submarine roll	8-inch long	60
Branola bread, wheat	2 slices	35
Bagel, Lender's	1 whole	30
English muffin, Thomas's	1 whole	27
Pita pocket	1 whole	33
Bran muffin	1 large	45
Pancakes, Aunt Jemima	2 × 4 inch	30
Waffle, Eggo	1	17
Matzo	1 sheet	28
Saltines	6	15
Graham crackers	1	10

Table 2-2 (continued)

Food	Amount	Carbohydrates (grams)
Granola bar, Nature Valley (cinnamon)	1 bar	17
Breakfast Cereals		
Grape-Nuts	¼ cup	23
Raisin Bran	½ cup	21
Granola, low-fat	¼ cup	18
Oatmeal, maple instant	1 packet	30
Cream of Wheat	1 serving	22
Beverages		
Apricot nectar	8 oz.	35
Cranberry-raspberry drink	8 oz.	36
Apple juice	8 oz.	29
Orange juice	8 oz.	27
Cola	12 oz.	38
Milk, chocolate	8 oz.	25
Milk, low-fat	8 oz.	12
Grains, Pasta, and Starches		
Baked potato	1 large	51
Stuffing	1 cup	40
Spaghetti, cooked	1 cup	40
Rice, cooked	1 cup	46
Ramen noodles	½ package	25
Legumes		
Baked beans	1 cup	50
Navy beans	1 cup	48
Black beans	1 cup	40
Lima beans	1 cup	32
Lentils, cooked	1 cup	40
Entrées, Convenience Foods		
Bean burrito	1	50
Chili	1 cup	45

Table 2-2 (continued)

Food	Amount	Carbohydrates (grams)
Macaroni and cheese	1 cup	45
Pizza, cheese	2 slices	42
Split pea soup	8 oz.	24
Sweets, Snacks, Desserts		
Maple syrup	2 tbsp.	25
Strawberry jam	1 tbsp.	13
Honey	1 tbsp.	15
Cranberry sauce	2 tbsp.	15
Fig Newtons	1	11
Chocolate chip cookie	1	10
Fruit yogurt	1 cup	50
Dairy Queen cone	1 medium	35

Fiber

Every time you crunch down on a piece of celery or bite into an apple, you're eating fiber, an indigestible but indispensable carbohydrate. Low amounts of fiber in the diet are linked to dozens of medical problems, including heart disease, cancer (especially colorectal cancer), diabetes, diverticulosis, and gallstones. See table 2-3 for a complete list.

Fiber is essential if you want to stay healthy and active as long as possible. There are two types of fiber, and their influence on risk factors for disease varies.

Water-Soluble Fiber

An indigestible remnant of food, fiber is classified by its ability to dissolve in water. Water-soluble fibers include plant material such as gums, mucilages, pectin, and some hemicelluloses. Gums and mucilages are sticky fibers proven to help regulate blood sugar and lower cholesterol. Pectin has a cholesterol-lowering effect, too. By binding to bile acids (a source of cholesterol in the body) in the intestines, pectin keeps cholesterol from recycling, thus reducing the body's total cholesterol pool. Hemicelluloses do their part by absorbing water in the digestive

Table 2-3

CONDITIONS AND DISEASES ASSOCIATED WITH POOR DIETARY FIBER INTAKE*

Appendicitis	Hemorrhoids
Cardiovascular disease	Hiatal hernia
Breast cancer	High blood pressure
Cholecystitis (inflammation of the	High cholesterol
gallbladder)	Ischemic heart disease
Colorectal cancer	Kidney stones
Constipation	Obesity
Coronary blood clotting	Ovarian cancer
Dental cavities	Peptic ulcer
Diabetes	Pyelonephritis (inflammation of the
Diverticulosis	kidney)
Gallstones	Stomach cancer
Gum disease	Varicose veins

*Note: No cause-and-effect relationship can yet be established.

tract and moving food faster through your system. These actions help relieve constipation, rid the body of cancer-causing substances, and assist in weight control.

Good sources of water-soluble fibers include barley, rice, corn, oats, legumes, apples, pears (especially the fleshy portions), citrus fruits, bananas, carrots, prunes, cranberries, seeds, and seaweed.

Water-Insoluble Fiber

Lignins, cellulose, and some hemicelluloses are water-insoluble fibers. Lignins usher bile acids and cholesterol out of the intestines. Cellulose, the roughage we tend to associate with fiber, acts like a stool softener and bulk former, improving elimination and flushing carcinogens from the system.

Good food sources of water-insoluble fibers include root and leafy vegetables, whole grains (such as wheat, barley, rice, corn, and oats), legumes, unpeeled apples and pears, and strawberries.

Fiber Requirements

How much fiber should you eat to get its protective benefits? The National Research Council recommends 20 to 35 g of fiber a day from both water-soluble and water-insoluble fiber. Most Americans get only about 11 g a day, however. If you're fiber-needy, try to increase your intake gradually. Doing so can help prevent

Table 2-4

COMMON FIBER-CONTAINING FOODS

Food	Portion	Dietary Fiber Content (in grams)
Kidney beans, cooked	¾ cup	9.3
Cereal, All-Bran	⅓ cup	8.5
Figs, dried	3 medium	7.2
Prunes, dried	3 medium	4.7
Pear	1 medium	4.1
Apple	1 large	4.0
Potato, baked with skin	1 medium	4.0
Banana	1 medium	3.8
Blackberries	½ cup	3.3
Carrots, cooked	½ cup	3.2
Barley, cooked	½ cup	3.0
Apple	1 small	2.8
Broccoli, cooked	½ cup	2.8
Strawberries	1 cup	2.8
Bread, whole wheat	1 slice	2.4
Cereal, wheat, flaked	¾ cup	1.8
Oatmeal, cooked	¾ cup	1.6
Apricots	3 medium	1.4
Peach	1 medium	1.3
Bread, white*	1 slice	0.6

*This entry is included for the sake of comparison.

Source: Compiled from manufacturer's data. From J. W. Anderson and S. R. Bridges, "Dietary Fiber Content of Selected Foods," *American Journal of Clinical Nutrition* 47 (1988): 440–447; and from J. Pennington and H. Church, *Bowes' and Church's Food Values of Portions Commonly Used,* 14th ed. (Philadelphia: J. B. Lippincott Company, 1985).

cramping, bloating, and other unpleasant symptoms often associated with increased fiber.

And, although a little is good, a lot is not necessarily better. Some studies suggest that excessive fiber in the diet decreases the absorption of calcium, iron, zinc, and other minerals. There's also a danger with using fiber supplements. Because the fiber passes through the intestinal tract undigested, large amounts consumed over a short time can form into a mass that can get lodged in the curves and bends of the small intestines. This can lead to an intestinal obstruction that only surgery can correct. It's far better to get your fiber from food rather than from supplements.

Finally, beware of misleading nutrition claims. "Fiber rich," "high fiber," and "good source of fiber" are commonly found on food ads and packages. But don't depend on such claims for your information. Read the "Nutrition Facts" on the label instead. A food should contain at least 2.5 to 3.0 g of dietary fiber per serving to qualify as a good source of fiber. In table 2-4, you'll find a list of common fiber-containing foods.

CHAPTER 3

Carbohydrates for Exercise and Competition

Fuel Sources during Exercise

When you're sitting around watching TV or reading a book, carbohydrates supply about 40 percent of your energy needs. But suppose you decide to lift some weights or take a hard run?

With strength training, you exert short bursts of effort, punctuated by a little rest between exercise sets. With exercise like this—or any high-intensity effort sustained for one to three minutes—carbohydrate (muscle glycogen) supplies about 95 percent of the fuel.

It's a slightly different story with aerobic exercise. During aerobic or endurance exercise, your body burns mainly carbohydrate and fat for fuel. With mild to moderate-intensity aerobics, say a light jog or fast walk, the fuel mix burned is about 50/50. Pick up the pace, and you'll burn more carbohydrate—as much as 80 percent. Initially the energy source is glucose circulating in the blood. At this higher level of intensity, especially at the beginning of exercise, it's just not as easy for the body to liberate fat for energy as it is stored carbohydrate. Mobilizing fat for the fuel mixture involves a series of complex chemical reactions requiring oxygen.

But as your heart starts pumping harder and more blood flows into tissues, oxygen is transported into cells. This means fat can be burned, too, since oxygen has to be present in cells for fat burning. Now that more oxygen is available, the fuel mixture for exercise starts changing. More fat and less carbohydrate are burned, especially with aerobic exercise lasting more than twenty minutes. After twenty minutes, fat is liberated from tissues and fat-burning enzymes start to kick in.

Eventually your oxygen-carrying capacity begins to drop off. Fatigued, the body reverts to using stored carbohydrate for energy. The more carbohydrate that's left in the muscles toward the end of exercise, the longer you can last. You generally store about 1,600 calories of glycogen in your muscles and liver. On average, about 1,200 calories of glycogen are stored in your muscles, and 400 calories in your liver.

The amount of glycogen stored in muscles is directly related to how much carbohydrate you eat and how well trained you are. Diets containing 60 to 65 percent or more of calories from carbohydrate allow for the greatest storage of glycogen in the muscles on a daily basis.

The more glycogen you store in your muscles, the longer you can train or work out. So to maintain your active lifestyle, your diet should always be high in carbohydrates.

How Carbohydrates Keep You Lean

Building lean muscle mass places high energy demands on the body. That's why energy-giving carbohydrates are absolutely essential to the muscle-making process. In fact, carbohydrates are the most important nutrient for building lean mass—and for helping the body *resist* fat gain. You need about 2,500 calories to manufacture a pound of lean muscle. The best nutrient to drive that muscle-building machinery is carbohydrate. It provides the most immediate, cleanest-burning source of power. The more muscle you have, the less flab you put on.

Athletes who live the high-carb lifestyle are among the leanest, most fit people I know. The carbohydrates they eat provide quick energy without demand for oxygen, specifically in short-burst activities such as strength training. Well-stocked with carbs, they can train all-out in their workouts and are thus able to maintain peak condition. Carbohydrates are also important for long-haul activities such as road races or marathons. If carb reserves in the liver or muscles become depleted, the body can't mobilize fats to keep going, and the runner "hits the wall." I know there has been a lot of talk recently about cutting carbs to lose body fat. Don't try that approach. Any time carbs are in short supply, you're apt to suffer fatigue. You certainly won't feel like working out! Eat carbs throughout the day, and you'll be amazed at your energy levels and by the progress you're making in your workouts.

Carbohydrates and Strength Training

I feel strongly that strength trainers should eat even more carbs than the standard 60 to 65 percent of total calories. To develop muscle, you must increase your calories, and the healthiest way to do that is to up your carb intake, not your intake of protein or fat. A good rule of thumb to remember is this: As calories increase, so should carbs.

Your strength-training performance will improve, too. Carbohydrates are valuable in short-burst, intense exercise like strength training because they give you the energy and stamina to push harder and longer for better results. If you're you the energy and stamina to push harder and longer for better results. If you're well loaded with carbs before your workout, plus take in some during your workout, you can go all out. Here's a case to support my point.

In one study, a group of strength trainers was fed a carbohydrate drink just before training and between exercise sets. Another group was given a placebo. For exercise, both groups did leg extensions at about 80 percent of their strength capacity, performing repeated sets of ten repetitions with rest between sets. What the researchers found was that the carbohydrate-fed group outlasted the placebo group, performing many more sets and reps.

Extra carbs give you the energy to work out hard and build body-firming muscle. Here's more proof: One group of bodybuilders ate a moderate-protein/high-carbohydrate diet in which 70 percent of the calories were from carbs. A second group followed a high-protein/low-carbohydrate diet in which 50 percent of the calories came from carbs. Before and after each diet, the researchers checked the subjects' muscular endurance (the ability to perform repeated contractions without fatiguing) in their leg muscles. The high-carbohydrate group kept going, whereas the low-carb subjects fizzled out early.

Carbohydrates and Cross Training

Cross training uses up a lot of muscle glycogen. Not replacing it will make you feel weak, and you won't have the power to push on in your exercise program.

To keep your energy tanks full, I recommend eating carbohydrates throughout the day—at breakfast, lunch, and dinner, along with two between-meal snacks. Try to include some protein each time you eat, too. The combination of carbohydrates and protein slows down your digestion a bit so that you don't get a fast surge of blood sugar from the carbs. Your energy level stays even throughout the day. One of the best snacks to eat is fruited yogurt, which is high in carbs and contains just enough protein for an even release of energy.

Right after exercise, you should recharge your muscles with carbs as soon as possible. In the first two hours following a workout, muscles are carb-needy, and they take up glucose fast. In chapter 16, you'll see how to use sports drinks to "mainline" glucose right to your muscles.

Carbohydrate Loading for Endurance Athletes

One of the few dietary methods known to make a real difference in physical performance, carbohydrate loading is a technique of pushing more glycogen into muscle storage than normal. Followed the week prior to competition, carbohydrate loading works best for endurance competitions lasting at least sixty to ninety minutes or more.

The basic strategy for carbohydrate loading is twofold: Rest your muscles prior to the race, and eat as much carbohydrate as you can. Both parts are important. Resting your muscles, then loading up on carbs, keeps your glycogen reserves well stocked in preparation for competition.

Seasoned athletes receive a bigger endurance payoff from carbohydrate loading than do beginners: The more well-trained you are, the greater your capacity to store glycogen. Even so, the technique helps the novice, too.

In the past, athletes tried to empty their glycogen stores, then load up on carbs just before the competition. This extreme, energy-sapping approach has been tossed out in favor of a better one. It achieves the same glycogen storage results, without leaving you irritable, tired, and sluggish the day before your race. Table 3-1 shows how to carbohydrate-load the right way.

A Precompetition Diet Plan

As shown in table 3-1, you should increase your carbs to 70 percent of your total calories the three days prior to competition. The following diet plan is an example of how to do this. A note of caution: Even though sweets and snack foods like desserts, crackers, and chips may have carbohydrate in them, they are usually too high in fat. Fat slows emptying from the stomach, creating discomfort and preventing the rapid use of nutrients. So stay away from fatty foods, especially just before a competition.

Breakfast
1½ cups whole grain cereal
1 cup skim milk
4 slices whole wheat toast or 2 bagels or 2 English muffins
2 tbsp. fruit spread
2 fresh fruit or fruit juice

Table 3-1

THE HIGH-PERFORMANCE CARBOHYDRATE-LOADING PLAN

Days Prior to Competition	Training Intensity	Diet
6	Flat out, hard—90 minutes	Usual diet, 60 to 65% carbs
5	Moderate—40 to 60 minutes	Usual diet, 60 to 65% carbs
4	Moderate—30 to 40 minutes	Usual diet, 60 to 65% carbs
3	Moderate—20 to 30 minutes	70% carbs; see the diet in the next section.
2	Light—20 minutes	70% carbs
1	Rest	70% carbs
Competition day	Go for it!	See following guidelines.

Snack
  3½ oz. dried fruit mix
Lunch
  2 water-packed tuna or turkey sandwiches on whole wheat bread
  2 tbsp. low-fat mayonnaise
  2 carrots
  2 fresh fruits or fruit juice
  2 Fig Newtons
Dinner
  2 cups brown rice
  1½ cups broccoli and chicken stir-fry
  2 cups green salad
  2 tbsp. reduced-calorie dressing
  1 fresh fruit
  1 cup frozen yogurt

Your Diet on Race Day

What you eat on race day makes a tremendous difference in your staying power. About two to three hours before the event, have a meal that's light and packed with carbs. Ideally, eat about 100 grams of carbs at this time. A combination of fruit, bread, rice, or pasta, with skim milk or nonfat yogurt, makes an excellent precompetition meal.

If you'd rather drink than eat, use a good high-carbohydrate sports drink such as GatorLode from Gatorade. This product—and others in the line—has been formulated according to the manufacturer's own published research. This research is peer reviewed by medical professionals working in the field of nutrition. Although I'm not endorsing Gatorade products, I place a lot of stock in the scientific credibility of their formulations and published effectiveness for physically active people. Other products might work best for you. Try them all.

Twenty to thirty minutes prior to the race, consume some additional carbs. But be careful! Eating too close to race time can cause blood sugar dips partway into competition. Stay away from candy bars—they're high in fat and will make you sluggish. The best plan is to drink a regular sports drink to help you with fluids as well as with carbs.

Carbohydrate Support during Competition

If you're competing in a long-endurance event, have some carbs in the form of a sports drink during your race. This helps stabilize your blood sugar levels, maintain fluid levels, and gives you extra pep. Research has consistently shown that drinking a sports drink during competition delays fatigue.

Drink a half cup of a regular sports drink every fifteen to twenty minutes to extend your endurance. The sports drink should contain a solution of 6 to 10 percent carbohydrate. This formulation empties from the stomach as quickly as plain water and delivers an appropriate concentration of easily digested and absorbed carbs to the working muscles.

Postevent Carbo- hydrates

Finally, after exercise, replenish your muscle glycogen stores. Following competition, your body starts making new glycogen within the first twenty-four hours, provided you start consuming sufficient dietary carbohydrate. Throughout the twenty-four hours just after competition, start eating or drinking high-carbohydrate foods, with 40 to 60 g of carbohydrate per hour for the first five hours of recovery. This is an especially important practice during repetitive competition trials and tournament play.

Staying Energetic

Whatever your sport or exercise, the single most important dietary factor affecting your performance is the amount of carbohydrate in your daily diet. Eating a high-carb diet regularly keeps your muscles well fueled so that you can challenge yourself physically and improve your performance during your regular workouts. Stick with carbs as the mainstay of your diet, and you won't believe how great you'll look, and how strong you'll feel.

CHAPTER 4

Fat

A Fuel Source

Along with carbohydrates, fat is an important fuel source for exercise and activity. Yet it is one nutrient we all seem to fear, especially since it's linked to the top three causes of death in this country—heart disease, cancer, and stroke. Even so, dietary fat is an essential nutrient, required to help form the structures of cell membranes, regulate metabolism, and provide a source of energy for exercise and activity.

The more scientists discover about fats, the more complex the story becomes. Ever-changing news on cholesterol and fats—which ones are good and which are bad—has made it nearly impossible to figure out what's healthy and relevant to active people, and what's not. Let's try to break the whole fat and cholesterol issue down to what you need to know to keep your performance level high.

Types of Dietary Fat

Most dietary fats are composed of triglycerides, a chemical combo of carbon, hydrogen, oxygen, and a type of alcohol called glycerol. During digestion, triglycerides are broken down into fatty acids and absorbed into the cells of the intestinal walls. The body wraps fatty acids in special protein blankets called lipoproteins. Lipoproteins help move fatty acids through the bloodstream. Metabolized by the body, lipoproteins are stored as fat, burned as energy, or used as building material for cell membranes.

Good and Bad Cholesterol

Lipoproteins contain cholesterol, an odorless, waxy fatlike substance found in all foods of animal origin. Needed for good health, cholesterol is a constituent of most body tissues. It's also used to make certain hormones, vitamin D, and bile. You don't need to consume cholesterol; your body makes enough all by itself.

If you overproduce cholesterol, the excess circulates in the bloodstream and collects in the inner walls of the arteries. Over time cholesterol accumulates in arteries like rust building up in pipes. This condition can lead to a heart attack.

The type of cholesterol responsible for depositing cholesterol in the artery walls is low-density lipoprotein, or LDL cholesterol. LDLs are known as "bad" cholesterol; the lower your blood values, the better.

High-density lipoprotein, or HDL cholesterol, is heart protective. Its job is to remove bad cholesterol from the cells in the artery wall and transport it back to the liver for reprocessing or excretion from the body as waste. HDLs are "good" cholesterol; the more in your blood, the better.

High blood cholesterol is a risk factor for heart disease that can be controlled. Have your cholesterol checked regularly by a blood analysis. The general recommendation for adults is to have an LDL level of below 130, an HDL level of 40 or above, and a total cholesterol reading of less than 200. If you have a cholesterol problem, follow your physician's orders.

Saturated and Unsaturated Fats

When it comes to raising cholesterol levels in the blood, dietary fat is clearly the biggest offender. But not all fat is to blame. Fatty acids are either *saturated* or *unsaturated,* terms that describe their chemical structure. Saturated fats are found mostly in beef, dairy products, commercially prepared baked goods, and tropical oils like coconut, palm, and palm kernel oils. These fats can raise LDL cholesterol to potentially dangerous levels.

Unsaturated fats aren't quite as bad. In fact, they contain key nutrients called essential fatty acids. Two of the most important are linoleic acid and linolenic acid, both found in vegetable oils. Essential fatty acids are required for normal growth, skin integrity, and healthy blood and nerves.

There are two types of unsaturated fats: polyunsaturated fats and monounsaturated fats. Vegetable oils such as safflower oil, sunflower oil, corn oil, soybean oil, and cottonseed oil are polyunsaturated fats.

Polyunsaturated fats cut cholesterol. But the problem is, they cut all cholesterol—the bad kind (LDL) and the good kind (HDL). To make matters worse, cancer researchers have discovered a close correlation between diets high in polyunsaturated fats and a greater risk of cancer.

Monounsaturated Fats

So what's a body to do? Enter the Eskimos and the Greeks. Even though their diets are high in total fat, their incidence of heart disease is low compared with Americans. Scientists have ascertained why: The predominant fat in both cultures is monounsaturated fat; in one culture from fish, in the other from olives.

Monounsaturated fats have a protective effect on blood cholesterol levels. They help lower the bad cholesterol but maintain higher levels of the good cholesterol. The Eskimos hit an even bigger nutritional jackpot than the Greeks: The fat in fish oils helps prevent blood clotting, a cause of strokes.

Clearly, you want monounsaturated fats in your diet. They're plentiful in olive oil, canola oil, and peanut oil, and in fish from cold waters, such as salmon, mackerel, halibut, swordfish, black cod, and rainbow trout, and in shellfish.

Hydroge-nated Fats

As for other dietary fats, watch out for foods containing hydrogenated vegetable oils and solid vegetable shortenings. These commercially processed unsaturated fats behave more like saturated fats. They're lower in polyunsaturated fatty acids and higher in saturated and monounsaturated fatty acids than the unhydrogenated versions of the same oils. Hydrogenated fats have been used in place of the saturated tropical oils in commercially baked products like crackers and cookies. But recent research indicates that hydrogenated fats may be more harmful in our diets than the tropical oils they replaced.

Controlling Fat Intake

By commandeering dietary fat, you may be able to delay or even prevent the life-threatening diseases linked to fat. To control fats strictly, you can monitor your fat intake in a number of ways. One involves eating adequate amounts of carbs. When working with clients, I always take the positive approach and stress the number of carb grams that should be eaten, rather than the number of fat grams that should be limited. By eating as many carbs as you can stand, you automatically eat less fat.

Calculating Your Daily Fat Intake

If you like numbers and calculations, you can monitor your fat intake by counting the grams of fat in your diet each day. Your daily fat intake should be 20 to 25 percent of your total calorie intake. That percentage should come mostly from monounsaturated fats and fish oils; second, from polyunsaturated fats; and last from saturated fats. A good rule of thumb to follow is 5 percent saturated fat, 8 percent monounsaturated fat, and 7 percent polyunsaturated fat.

You can calculate your own daily fat intake by using the following formulas:

Step 1: Total fat: Total calories × 20% = daily calories from fat ÷ 9 – _____ grams total fat. (For example: 2,000 calories × .20 = 400 ÷ 9 = 44 g total fat.)

Step 2: Saturated fatty acids (SFA): Total calories × 5% = daily calories from SFA ÷ 9 = _____ grams SFA. (For example: 2,000 calories × .05 = 100 ÷ 9 = 11 g SFA.)

Read Food Labels for Fat Content

Once you've calculated your own dietary allowance for total fat and saturated fat, read food labels for the fat content per serving. The grams of fat are listed under "Nutrition Facts" on any food package that provides a nutrition label.

Another way to monitor your fat intake is by limiting the majority of foods in your diet to those that have only 25 percent or less of their calories from fat. By using the information on the nutrition label, you can easily determine whether a food meets this criterion. Use the following formula to find percentage of calories from fat:

$$\frac{\text{calories of fat per serving}}{\text{total calories per serving}}$$

Suppose an item of food has 36 fat calories in a serving, and the total calories per serving are 220. Here's an example using that label information:

$$\frac{36 \text{ fat calories}}{220 \text{ calories per serving}} = .16 \times 100 = 16\% \text{ of calories from fat}$$

Healthy Fat Choices

By eating a diet high in vegetables, fruits, grains, and beans and using the healthy oils suggested, you'll automatically tend toward the healthiest ratio of fats in your diet. Choose margarines that have a liquid oil as the first ingredient. Use low-fat and skim milk dairy products, and eat mostly fish, seafood, and skinless poultry and small portions of beef.

A word about butter versus margarine: I use very little solid fat in my diet, but when I do, my choice is butter. I like the taste better, and it may be healthier than margarine. Margarine contains substances called trans fatty acids that appear to impair cardiovascular health. As noted above, if you like margarine, choose a product that has a liquid oil as the first ingredient. Limit your intake of margarine, however, to control the total amount of fat in your diet.

Fat as a Fuel Source for Exercisers

Fat in the form of fatty acids is burned during exercise, along with carbohydrates. The longer and harder you can exercise aerobically, the more fat you'll burn. Aerobic training in particular increases the activity of fat-burning enzymes in cells, and these start working once you exceed twenty minutes of aerobic exercise. The cells then become more efficient in burning fatty acids drawn from body fat stores and rely less on muscle glycogen. The more aerobically fit you are, the better you can burn fat. Highly trained endurance athletes are able to tap into fat stores for energy, saving muscle glycogen for the latter stages of competition.

Fat Loading

The role of fat in providing energy for endurance exercise has prompted researchers to investigate whether elevating fats in the diet spares carbohydrates from being used for energy and thus improves performance. The practice has become known as "fat loading." I've got my doubts about it, but let's take a look at what one study shows.

Researchers compared a high-carb, fat-restricted diet with a moderate-carb, fat-rich diet on running performance. Six college runners were tested on three different diets: a high-fat diet (50 percent carbs, 38 percent fat, and 12 percent protein); a high-carb, low-fat diet (73 percent carbs, 15 percent fat, and 12 percent protein); and a normal diet (61.2 percent carbs, 24.3 percent fat, and 13.7 percent protein). The runners performed best on the fat-rich diet and worst when fat was restricted on the high-carb diet.

Experiments with experienced runners are one thing, but what about regular exercisers or weekend athletes? Can they work out harder and longer by eating more fat? The answer is no. Remember, one study never tells the whole story. Plus, the study has not yet been repeated, nor does it apply to the larger population.

In fact, high-fat foods should be avoided in the twelve-hour period before exercise. The reason is, high-fat foods increase fatty acids in the blood. This elevation triggers the release of a brain chemical called serotonin, which causes sleepiness and fatigue. More important, too much fat in the diet is unhealthy and can greatly compromise your potential for an active lifetime.

CHAPTER 5

Protein

The Function of Protein in the Body

Protein is a nutrient essential to physical performance and high-level health because of its role in growth and maintenance. Like carbohydrates and fat, protein is a chemical structure containing carbon, hydrogen, and oxygen. The only difference is that protein has one other element—nitrogen. At the molecular level, protein is made up of smaller units called amino acids, which are connected together like a strand of pearls. If two strands of pearls were wound together, and then twisted to double up on each other, they'd resemble a protein molecule.

Your body breaks down dietary protein into amino acids and reshuffles them into new protein to build and rebuild tissue, including muscle. Protein also keeps your immune system functioning up to par, helps carry nutrients throughout the body, has a hand in forming hormones, and is involved in important enzyme reactions such as digestion.

There are twenty different types of amino acids, and all can be combined to form the proteins necessary to build the body and keep it healthy. Some of these amino acids can be made by the body and are called nonessential, or dispensable, amino acids. Others have to be supplied by the foods you eat. These amino acids are termed essential, or indispensable, amino acids. Animal and plant foods contain all twenty amino acids, but in different amounts depending on the food. Animal proteins are of a higher quality because they contain all the essential amino acids in larger amounts and better proportions. In plants, amino acids exist in smaller concentrations. For the body to make protein properly, all twenty amino acids must be present at the same time.

Although amino acids work together to form body proteins, individual amino acids have specific roles to play in the body. Certain amino acids such as tryptophan and tyrosine are involved in the formation of chemical messengers called neurotransmitters for the brain. A trio of amino acids (leucine, isoleucine, and valine), technically known as the branched-chain amino acids, are constituents of muscle tissue.

Protein and Energy

Is protein ever an energy source? Yes and no. If you eat too much protein, the excess can be converted to carbohydrate to be used for energy or to fat for storage. In diets that overly restrict calories, carbohydrates, and fats, the body starts burning protein for energy, since energy production takes metabolic priority over tissue building. But protein is underemployed in this job. Using protein as an energy source is like hiring a computer specialist, then relegating him or her to the mailroom. Protein has more important jobs to do in the body than supply energy.

There's one major exception, however. We now know that certain amino acids—the branched-chain amino acids—are used for energy in endurance exercise lasting at least sixty to ninety minutes. During high-intensity aerobic exercise, one branched-chain amino acid in particular—leucine—is rapidly used up. The by-products of its breakdown are used to make another amino acid called alanine, which the liver converts to glucose. Eventually that glucose finds its way to the working muscles and is used for energy. The harder you work out aerobically, the more leucine you use. This major new finding sheds light on why hard-training endurance athletes use amino acids for energy production.

Do Strength Trainers Need More Protein?

Because of protein's role in forming lean muscle tissue, it's no wonder that protein has long been touted as the food of athletes, particularly strength athletes such as bodybuilders, weight lifters, and football players. The first account of someone using a high-protein diet and strength training to build muscle and strength dates back to antiquity with the story of Milo, a champion wrestler who was the victor in five Olympic games. Every day Milo carried a growing calf the length of the Olympic stadium. As the calf grew progressively heavier, eventually maturing into a cow, Milo's strength increased exponentially. And it was believed that Milo ate 20 pounds of meat a day. With Milo, the myth was born that eating extra protein gives you greater muscular strength.

For generations, iron-pumping enthusiasts have stood by protein as the nutritional answer to muscle building. Only recently have scientists put this gym talk to the test, and there's now convincing proof that bodybuilders, weight lifters, and other strength athletes may have been right all along. As a strength trainer, you benefit from eating some extra protein. Here are a few cases that support my point:

> ✔ At Tufts University, elderly subjects who supplemented their diets with extra protein while following a strength-training program gained much more muscle mass than a control group who did not supplement while strength-training. The researchers did CAT scans, a high-tech imaging technique, to view the amount of muscle gained.

✔ A similar study looked into the effects of extra protein on young subjects engaged in a four-week bodybuilding program. Two groups of these young bodybuilders followed the same diet, but with one exception. One group ate 2.3 g of protein per kilogram of body weight (a very large amount), compared with 1.3 g of protein in the control group. By the end of the study, both groups had put on muscle. But those eating the higher amount of protein had gained *five times more muscle!*

✔ At Kent State University, researchers divided people into three groups of strength trainers. Each group was categorized as follows: a low-protein group on a diet of .9 g of protein per kilogram of body weight, which approximates the protein requirement for sedentary people; a group eating 1.4 g of protein per kilogram of body weight; and a group eating 2.4 g of protein. The study also had controls, both sedentary subjects and strength-training subjects. Two exciting findings emerged. First, increasing protein intake to 1.4 g triggered protein synthesis (an indicator of muscle growth) in strength-training individuals. No such changes occurred in the low-protein group. Second, upping protein intake from 1.4 g to 2.4 g produced no further protein synthesis. This latter finding suggested that a plateau had been reached, meaning that the subjects got more protein than they could use at 2.4 g.

Clearly, if you strength-train and eat more protein, you're going to enhance muscle development and preservation. But does this mean you should start loading up on protein-rich foods? Not necessarily. Let's talk about how much protein you really need for your individual activity level.

Calculating Your Daily Protein Requirements

If You Don't Work Out

If you're a sedentary adult—that is, you don't exercise or get much activity—the recommended dietary allowance (RDA) for protein is .36 g per pound of body weight per day. To calculate your protein requirement, multiply your weight in pounds by .36 g. Here's how to figure that requirement if you weigh 150 lb.:

.36 g of protein per pound of body weight × 150 lb. =
54 g of protein a day.

If You Strength- Train

You *do* need extra protein when you're working out, and the requirements differ slightly, depending on how you exercise. If you strength-train regularly (and I hope you do), you need .7 g of protein per pound of body weight a day. Using the preceding example again:

.7 g of protein per pound of body weight × 150 lb. =
105 g of protein a day.

Table 5-1

GOOD SOURCES OF PROTEIN

Food	Amount	Protein (grams)
Animal Foods		
Beef, lean	4 oz.	24
Chicken breast	3 oz.	24
Fish	3 oz	16–18
Turkey, light meat	4 oz.	9
Dairy Products		
Cheese	1 oz.	8
Cottage cheese, 2%	½ cup	16
Egg	1 large	6
Egg white	1 large	4
Milk, dried nonfat, instant	1 cup	24
Milk, low-fat	1 cup	8
Milk, skim	1 cup	8
Yogurt, low-fat, plain	8 oz.	12
Yogurt, low-fat, fruit	8 oz.	11
Nuts, Seeds, & Nut Products		
Peanuts	1 oz.	7
Peanut butter	2 tbsp.	8
Pumpkin seeds	½ cup	20
Sunflower seeds	1 tbsp.	3
Soy Products		
Soybeans, cooked	½ cup	14
Soy milk	1 cup	8
Tofu	½ cup	20
Vegetables/High-Protein		
Beans, black	½ cup	8
Beans, pinto	½ cup	7
Chickpeas (garbanzos)	½ cup	20
Lentils	½ cup	9

If You Do Aerobics

If you do aerobics only, your requirement is lower—.5 g of protein per pound of body weight:

$$.5 \text{ g of protein per pound of body weight} \times 150 \text{ lb.} =$$
$$75 \text{ g of protein a day.}$$

If You're an Endurance Athlete or a Cross Trainer

Those of you who perform hard endurance exercise and cross-train with intense strength training may need as much as .9 g of protein per pound of body weight. Here's the math:

$$.9 \text{ g of protein per pound of body weight} \times 150 \text{ lb.} =$$
$$135 \text{ g of protein a day.}$$

A Healthy Amount of Protein

As far as the composition of your diet is concerned, make sure that about 15 percent of your total calories comes from protein. You should have no trouble getting enough protein from foods. (See table 5-1 for a look at the number of grams in protein foods.) In fact, most active people, exercisers or athletes, on healthy diets rarely need to increase their protein intake. Usually they're eating too much protein.

This brings up another key point about protein: An excess in the system can be bad news. When protein molecules are disassembled during metabolism, the nitrogen portion is snipped off. Extra nitrogen floating around in the body is a poison that has to be detoxified. In the process, an intermediary toxin is created—ammonia. Eventually ammonia is turned into harmless urea and excreted. A system overloaded in this manner can endanger the kidneys in people susceptible to kidney problems.

Also, a diet too high in protein may cause kidney cancer, according to new research from the National Cancer Institute. Scientists there analyzed the diets of 690 kidney cancer patients and found that people whose diets included large amounts of meat, eggs, milk, cheese, and cereals were 90 percent more likely to get kidney tumors than those who ate modest amounts of protein. This is certainly an intriguing study, although it's too soon to say exactly what impact the study will have on nutrition and cancer research.

CHAPTER 6

Phytochemicals

What Are Phytochemicals?

Picture a bed of green, leafy lettuce piled high with carrots, onions, tomato, broccoli, and cabbage. A few ounces of tofu are crumbled on for protein. The salad is drizzled with a dressing made from flaxseed oil with some chopped garlic thrown in for flavor. This crispy, palate-pleasing meal is dishing out a lot more than vitamins, minerals, and fiber. You're about to eat of plateful of "phytochemicals."

Sound unappetizing? Don't let the name scare you. Nature has given us a virtual cornucopia of health-giving nutrients in our foods. Now scientists have discovered some new components in foods that have some amazing disease-fighting properties. They're called *phytochemicals,* which means plant chemicals.

Phytochemicals in Your Diet

The food you eat contains thousands of these chemicals. This is good news to athletes and exercisers because most phytochemicals are found in carbohydrate-containing foods, the main source of energy during exercise. If you're eating plenty of carbs, you're getting a healthy dose of phytochemicals.

Unlike vitamins and minerals, phytochemicals are not nutrients, but they do seem to protect against cancer, heart disease, and other illnesses. For more than twenty years, scientists have known that people who eat a lot of fruits, vegetables, and grains have lower rates of most cancers. In 1989 Herbert F. Pierson, a toxicologist who was working at the National Cancer Institute at the time, started studying the naturally occurring substances in these foods to better understand how they protect against cancer. What he found was that many of these substances exert subtle druglike effects and influence the body's biochemistry in positive ways.

How Phytochemicals Work

Let's return to the salad for a moment and pick it apart, ingredient by ingredient, so you can see what phytochemicals mean to your health.

First, the garlic and onions contain phytochemicals called allylic sulfides. These have been shown in the lab to inhibit tumor production. Like a football player intercepting a pass, compounds in garlic catch carcinogens before they can attack genetic material in cells and cause disease. Allylic sulfides have been linked to lower rates of stomach cancer.

Vegetables such as broccoli and cabbage contain sulforaphane and indoles. In lab animals, sulforaphane appears to prevent breast cancer. When added to live human cells in a lab dish, sulforaphane activated the production of special enzymes that ward off cancer.

Indoles are another phytochemical in these vegetables. They go to work against dangerously high levels of estrogen, potentially reducing the risk of breast cancer. Cauliflower, brussels sprouts, and kohlrabi contain sulforaphane and indoles, too.

One of the better-studied phytochemicals, beta-carotene, is found in carrots and gives the vegetable its characteristic orange color. Beta-carotene is an antioxidant nutrient, known to thwart a normal metabolic process called oxidation. Oxidation produces free radicals, unstable molecules that cause irreversible damage to cell membranes. Antioxidants step in and stop this cellular havoc. (For more information on antioxidants and free radicals, see chapters 7, 8, and 9).

Tomatoes have as many as ten thousand phytochemicals in them. One of the most important is lycopene, an antioxidant that may help prevent heart disease and cancer. Others are p-coumaric acid and chlorogenic acid. During digestion, both acids interfere with the production of nitrosamines, compounds of nitric acid and protein particles called amines. The tomato acids come along and steal the nitric acid from cells before it can bond to amines. Nitrosamines have been implicated in the development of stomach cancer.

The flaxseed-based salad dressing is rich in alpha-linolenic acid, which is converted into an omega-3 fatty acid. Omega-3 fats are inflammation fighters and may help prevent heart disease.

Phytoestrogens

Tofu and other soy-based products are packed with phytochemicals called phytoestrogens. During a woman's childbearing years, these natural chemicals help prevent breast cancer by competing with naturally occurring estrogens in the body. In menopause, estrogen production drops by 60 percent. Phytoestrogens can help make up the difference but without increasing the risk of cancer.

Evidence of the power of phytoestrogens can be seen among people who eat a lot of soy foods. Asian women, for example, eat low-fat diets with large amounts of tofu and other soy-based products. They have five times less the rate of breast cancer than women who eat a typical Western diet. When breast cancer does strike Asian women, it takes a more favorable course, with a higher cure rate.

The most important phytoestrogens now making their mark in nutrition are isoflavones, especially genistein and daidzein.

Isoflavones

Isoflavones look and act like the female sex hormone estrogen. But compared with natural estrogen, they are much weaker—only about one hundred-thousandth as strong. Even so, they appear to help prevent the abnormal activity of estrogen, a long-accepted link to breast cancer. Most breast cancers are estrogen dependent, meaning estrogen fuels their growth. High levels of estrogen have been linked to a greater risk of breast cancer and other hormone-needy cancers.

For estrogen to work, it has to gain entry into cells by first attaching to receptors on cell membranes. These receptors are like door buzzers signaling the cell to open up and let certain substances in. Estrogen and isoflavones seem to compete with each other on the doorstep of the cell membrane. Like two visitors ringing the same buzzer, they vie for entry into the cell. In doing so, isoflavones keep estrogen from attaching to the receptors and doing its job. This mix-up blocks estrogen from entering cells, possibly reducing the risk of breast cancer.

Isoflavones appear to have a split personality. In premenopausal women, who have a lot of circulating estrogen, isoflavones cause the body to produce less of the hormone. Yet they work just the opposite way in postmenopausal women, who have low levels of the hormone. After menopause, estrogen production falls off. This time, there's less estrogen on the cell's doorstep. Isoflavones have no problem hooking up to the receptors and getting inside the cell, where they increase levels of estrogen.

Among other physiological functions, estrogen controls a woman's menstrual cycle. It's well known that longer menstrual cycles are linked to a lower risk of breast cancer. In one study, women ate soy daily for two months to see whether the length of their menstrual cycles changed in any way. As it turned out, in five of the six women, their cycles increased by two and a half days. When isoflavones were removed from the soy product used in the study, there was no change in the length of the women's cycles. The researchers concluded that isoflavones exerted some powerful physiological effects.

Men shouldn't feel left out. Because of phytoestrogens' regulating action on hormones, they may help prevent prostate cancer, another hormone-dependent cancer. Scientists also feel that isoflavones and lignan, another phytochemical in soy foods, may directly inhibit the growth and spread of hormone-needy cancer cells.

Genistein   The isoflavone genistein is making news. In fact, genistein has generated so much excitement that the number of scientific papers published on it doubled each year between 1985 and 1993. In test tubes, genistein inhibits the growth of cancer cells, but not normal cells. The list of cancer cells thwarted by genistein is growing, too: breast, colon, lung, prostrate, skin, and leukemia.

It's too early to tell what genistein does to these cells in the body, but scientists do know that it interferes with the growth of blood vessels that feed tumors. When these supply routes are cut off, tumors can't get the oxygen and nutrients they need to grow. Because genistein deters tumor growth in this manner, it may someday become valuable in both the prevention and treatment of cancer. Also, genistein appears to protect against high cholesterol.

Daidzein   Daidzein is an isoflavone in soy foods that may actually promote bone building. Soy foods cause less calcium to be excreted in urine, and scientists think daidzein may be the reason, although it's too early to know for sure. But if so, eating soy foods could be another shield against osteoporosis.

Eat More Soy Foods

A good move is to include more soy products in your diet, particularly as substitutes for meat or milk in low-fat cooking. Be aware, however, that the phytoestrogen content of soy foods varies from product to product. A recent study from

Table 6-1

SOURCES AND FUNCTIONS OF PHYTOCHEMICALS

Phytochemicals	Food Source	Protective Action
Alpha-linolenic acid	Flaxseed oil	Converts into an omega-3 fatty acid, which acts as an anti-inflammatory agent and may also protect against heart disease
Allylic sulfides	Garlic, onions, and leeks	Usher carcinogens from the body; decrease tumor reproduction; and fortify the immune system
Capsaicin	Hot peppers	Prevents toxic molecules from latching on to genetic material in cells
Casseic acid	Fruits	Helps the body produce an enzyme that rids the body of carcinogens
Carotenoids	Orange and yellow vegetables	Prevent damage to cell membranes and to genetic material inside cells
Ellagic acid	Grapes	Prevents toxic chemicals from damaging cells
Ferulic acid	Fruits	Binds to nitrites in foods to prevent them from turning into carcinogenic substances called nitrosamines
Flavonoids	Citrus fruits	Detoxify dangerous chemicals; regulate enzymes to keep cells from becoming cancerous
Genistein	Soybeans	Prevents the formation of blood vessels that feed tumors. Inhibits platelet aggregation and reduces cholesterol for a heart-protective effect.

Table 6-1 (continued)

Phytochemicals	Food Source	Protective Action
Glucarates	Apples	Help rid the body of hormones that are linked to breast and prostate cancers
Indoles	Broccoli, cauliflower, cabbage, brussels sprouts, and kohlrabi	Help deactivate estrogen, a hormone linked to breast cancer
Isoflavones	Soybeans	Prevent blood vessels from forming in tumors, blocking their growth
Isothiocyanate	Horseradish	Activates an antioxidant enzyme called glutathione, which detoxifies carcinogens
Lignans	Flaxseed	Exerts antiestrogenic activity, reducing the risk of breast cancer
Limonene	Oranges	Stops damaged cells from uncontrolled growth
Lycopene	Tomatoes	Protects against heart disease and cancer
P-coumaric acid and chlorogenic acid	Tomatoes	Prevent the formation of carcinogens called nitrosamines during digestion.
Phenolics	Citrus fruits	Neutralize carcinogens and stimulate the production of glutathione, a detoxifying enzyme
Phytates	Grains	Bind to iron, possibly halting the formation of carcinogenic free radicals
Phytoestrogens	Tofu and soy products	Regulate healthy balances of estrogen, providing protection against breast cancer
Protease inhibitors	Legumes and dried beans	Retard the activity of certain enzymes in cancer cells to slow tumor growth
Saponins	Onions	Lower blood pressure, reduce cholesterol, and prevent cancer cells from multiplying
Sulforaphane	Broccoli, cauliflower, cabbage, brussels sprouts, and kohlrabi	Protects cells against carcinogens
Tannins	Green tea	Lower blood pressure, reduce cholesterol, and reduce the risk of esophageal cancer
Triterpenoids	Licorice root	Prevent tooth decay and reduce the risk of breast cancer

Tufts University School of Medicine showed that tofu contains high amounts of the isoflavones genistein and daidzein, but the content varies slightly among brands. Some dietary supplements formulated from what's known as "isolated soy protein" contain no phytoestrogens at all. Read labels to be sure of what you're getting.

Twenty-six Phytochemicals and Their Functions

Now that so many phytochemicals have been discovered, there are good reasons for multiple trips to the salad bar. Some scientists envision a day when foods will be fortified with phytochemicals. Until then you can get all the disease-fighting power of phytochemicals by simply eating a variety of fruits, vegetables, and grains—and lots of them—every day.

There are phytochemicals yet to be discovered—all the more reason to eat whole foods. Table 6-1 lists twenty-six of the more widely studied phytochemicals and their many remarkable functions.

CHAPTER 7

Vitamins

Energy-Releasing Nutrients

The joy of the high-performance life is a superfit body—vital, energetic, and able to withstand disease. Along with an active lifestyle, one of the ways to get a superfit body is by eating a variety of whole foods every day—carbs, protein, and a little bit of essential fat. Every time you pile these nutrients on your plate, you're serving up a lot more than meets the eye. The foods you eat are chock-full of thousands of unseen compounds, including vitamins. Among other functions, vitamins play a key role in releasing energy from foods so that you can maintain high-performance levels.

RDAs and What They Mean

No doubt you've heard the term *RDA,* which stands for Recommended Dietary Allowance. Established in 1943 by the government's National Research Council, the RDAs first served as a guide for advising the military on nutrition problems related to national defense. Since then they've been used in many other ways, from planning diets for specific groups of people to formulating new food products.

Revised periodically by nutrition scientists, the RDAs set forth eighteen essential micronutrients (vitamins and minerals) in specified amounts that you and I need for good nutritional health. Many experts, however, contend that the RDAs in their present form are too low for some groups of people, namely the elderly and the very active. Additionally it's been argued that the disease-preventing recommendations for vitamins A, E, and C, as well as fiber, aren't adequately addressed by the RDAs. Both arguments have some validity, although the RDA Committee says more research is needed before requirements are bumped up.

For now, the RDAs are the main yardstick by which nutritional intake is measured, even though some strong data support changes in this standard. Tables 7-1

Table 7-1

FACTS ABOUT VITAMINS

Vitamin	Exercise-Related Function	Beneficial Effects in Aging	Best Food Sources	Side Effects and Toxicity	RDA for Adults
Vitamin B Complex					
Thiamin (B$_1$)	Carbohydrate metabolism; maintenance of a healthy nervous system; growth and muscle tone	None known	Brewer's yeast, wheat germ, bran, whole grains, and organ meats	None known	0.5 mg per 1,000 calories consumed
Riboflavin (B$_2$)	Metabolism of carbohydrate, protein, and fat; cellular respiration	May help prevent cataracts	Milk, eggs, lean meats, and broccoli	None known	1.2 mg
Pyridoxine (B$_6$)	Protein metabolism; formation of oxygen-carrying red blood cells	Required for the production of antibodies	Whole grains and meats	Liver and nerve damage	1.6 mg
Cyanocobalamin (B$_{12}$)	Metabolism of carbohydrate, protein, and fat; formation of red blood cells	May help protect against heart disease	Meats, dairy products, eggs, liver, and fish	Liver damage, allergic reactions	2 µg
Niacin	Cellular energy production; metabolism of carbohydrates, protein, and fat	Improves circulation and reduces cholesterol levels in the blood; may be cancer protective	Lean meats, liver, poultry, fish, peanuts, and wheat germ	Liver damage, jaundice, skin flushing and itching, nausea	18 mg for men; 13 mg for women

Folic acid	Regulation of growth; breakdown of proteins; formation of red blood cells; protection against neurological defects in newborns	Helps prevent precancerous changes in the uterus; may protect against heart disease	Green leafy vegetables and liver	Gastric problems; can mask certain anemias	200 µg; 180 µg during pregnancy
Biotin	Breakdown of fats	None known	Egg yolks and liver	None known	30–100 µg
Pantothenic acid	Cellular energy production; fatty acid oxidation	Required for the production of antibodies; helps prevent premature aging	Found widely in foods	None known	4–7 mg
Vitamin A	Growth and repair; building of body structures	Maintenance of good eyesight; may reduce the risk of certain cancers and protect heart health	Liver, egg yolks, whole milk, and orange and yellow vegetables	Digestive system upset; damage to bones and certain organs	5,000 IU
Vitamin D	Normal bone growth and development	May help prevent osteoporosis	Sunlight, fortified dairy products, and fish oils	Nausea, vomiting, hardening of soft tissues, kidney damage	200 IU
Vitamin K	Involved in glycogen formation and blood clotting	Involved in normal liver functioning	Vegetables, milk, and yogurt	Allergic reactions, breakdown of red blood cells.	1 µg per kg of body weight

and 7-3 show the RDAs for various types of vitamins, along with their benefits and functions in the body.

How Vitamins Work

I could fill an entire book on vitamins alone, since most of them have been well researched and well publicized. Vitamins are required by the body in tiny amounts, compared with the requirements for carbohydrate, protein, and fat. Vitamins don't provide energy but instead trigger many energy-producing reactions in the body.

There are thirteen different vitamins, separated into two classes: water-soluble (B vitamins and vitamin C) and fat-soluble (vitamins A, D, E, and K). Fat-soluble vitamins, which require fat to be transported and used, are held in storage until needed somewhere in the body. The liver, for example, stocks a huge supply of vitamin A, sending it out to organs and tissues on request. Water-soluble vitamins, on the other hand, are not as easily stored. A nutritional liability of vitamins is that they're easily destroyed by food preparation, handling, and cooking. Table 7-2 provides guidelines on how to minimize this loss.

Upon entering the body, a vitamin travels through the bloodstream to the cells, where it joins up with enzymes to do its job. The cells can only use so much of the vitamin. When a certain ceiling is reached, several things can happen. The vitamin might be excreted if it's a water-soluble vitamin or stored if it's a fat-soluble vitamin. In certain situations, it may start acting like a drug, rather than as a nutrient. Taking vitamins over and above requirements doesn't serve any useful purpose and, in some cases, may be harmful.

B Vitamins and Exercisers

The B-complex vitamins, eleven in all, have been widely promoted as pepper-uppers for exercisers, since they help convert food to fuel. Riboflavin, plentiful in milk, can be easily sweated away during vigorous exercise. So can thiamin, especially with high-intensity endurance activities. Excessive alcohol use, calorie-restrictive diets, and nutrient-poor diets that are high in fat and refined sugar can also deplete thiamin.

Does this mean you should take some extra Bs to keep from pooping out? Not necessarily—unless you're an erratic eater, an alcoholic, or someone who often gorges on a lot of high-fat, refined foods. Then you could fall into the clutches of a vitamin B deficiency. However, dietary requirements for the B-complex group can be easily met if you eat a nutrient-rich diet, with the right proportion of quality carbs, protein, and essential fats to fuel your energy needs. As for boosting exercise stamina, some studies have looked into the effect of vitamin B supplementation but have failed to produce much firm justification for its use.

Table 7-2

SAVING THE VITAMINS IN YOUR VEGGIES

Certain nutrients are very sensitive to exposure to heat, light, water, and oxygen. No matter how careful you are with your cooking methods, cooking of any kind destroys nutrients or causes them to leach out from the food. After you've diligently planned your diet, you'll want to preserve the nutrient content of your food by following these guidelines:

1. Buy fresh produce that is crisp and not wilted. Avoid buying precut produce. If you can't shop often enough to keep produce fresh, opt for frozen vegetables. They're as high in nutrients as fresh food.

2. Keep skins on or keep produce well wrapped and sealed during refrigeration. Do not soak fruits or vegetables.

3. The peels of fruits and vegetables help prevent nutrient loss. Scrub produce well, then cook it whole or in large chunks.

4. Quick cooking methods, at high temperatures with the least exposure to water, preserve the greatest amount of nutrients. Stir-frying, microwaving, grilling, and steaming are the preferable cooking methods.

5. Cook foods for the shortest amount of time possible.

6. If cooking in water, use small amounts just to cover the food, and cover pots or pans to speed the cooking time.

7. Always make sure the cooking temperature is reached before adding the food. Return the water to boil as quickly as possible after the food has been added.

8. Cook veggies until just soft but still crisp and colorful.

9. Serve food promptly.

Vitamins A, D, and K

The fat-soluble vitamins A, D, and K are rarely promoted as exercisers' aids, most likely because they're toxic in large doses. Found in yellow and orange vegetables and some fish oils, vitamin A is involved in the growth and repair of tissues, maintenance of proper vision, and resistance to infection. It also helps maintain the health of the skin and mucous membranes. Massive doses in excess of the RDA can cause nausea, vomiting, diarrhea, skin problems, and bone fragility, among other serious problems.

Obtained mainly from sunlight and fortified dairy products, vitamin D helps your body absorb calcium and break down phosphorus, a mineral required for bone formation. Too much vitamin D causes serious changes in the body, including calcium loss and hardening of the soft tissues of organs.

Vitamin K's main job is the production of prothrombin, a chemical required in blood clotting. You get vitamin K naturally from green leafy vegetables, milk, vegetable oils, and fish oils. Too much of this vitamin causes serious blood problems, including anemia.

The Antioxidant Vitamins and Free Radicals

Certain vitamins, namely vitamin C, vitamin E, and beta-carotene, are called antioxidants because they protect the body against disease-causing substances known as free radicals. Free radicals are highly reactive molecules that tote around an extra electron. Like someone frantic to find a mate, they pair up with electrons of other molecules and claim them as their own. This causes harmful reactions in the body, particularly to cell membranes. Cell membranes become pitted, making it easy for bacteria, viruses, and other disease-causing agents to slip inside cells and do their dirty work. It's been estimated that cells sustain more than ten thousand free radical hits a day! Free radicals can destroy cells, tissues, even organs, weakening the immune system and leaving the body vulnerable to cancer and other diseases.

Free Radicals and Exercise

Many factors give rise to these biological troublemakers, including normal metabolism, aging, stress, sunlight, and exposure to environmental toxins such as cigarette smoke, exhaust fumes, and other pollutants. Exercise also generates free radicals. Scientists have discovered that hard-training athletes, specifically endurance and ultraendurance athletes, often have low levels of antioxidants circulating in their bodies, possibly due to free radical activity.

We don't know how or why exercise does this, but there are some theories. One has to do with respiration, the sum total of all the processes associated with the release of energy in the body. During respiration, cells pick off electrons from sugars and add them to oxygen to generate energy. As these reactions take place, electrons sometimes get off course and collide with other molecules, creating free radicals. By exercising, you step up respiration, and this produces more free radicals. It gets fairly chaotic at the cellular level.

Body temperature, which tends to rise during exercise, may also be a factor in generating free radicals. A third possibility is the increase in catecholamine production during exercise. Catecholamines are hormones released in response to muscular effort. They increase heart rate, let more blood get to muscles, and provide the muscles with fuel, among other functions. The point is, several complex reactions occur with exercise, and each one may accelerate free radical production.

Now you're probably thinking exercise isn't such a good deal after all. Before you jump to that conclusion, let me assure you that the benefits of exercise definitely outweigh the risks. The Centers for Disease Control (CDC) in Atlanta estimates that 250,000 people die each year because they don't get regular exercise. Remember: Exercise combined with high-performance nutrition keeps your body tuned to high-performance levels all day.

The Role of Antioxidant Vitamins

Nutritionally, we need something to foil the free radical rampage going on inside our bodies. That's where antioxidant vitamins come in. They're the body's own natural cleanup crew. They scour free radicals from the body and prevent new ones from being formed.

Free radicals normally don't cause much of a problem. As long as you're healthy and functioning up to par, the antioxidant cleanup crew is at work, taking care of free radicals. But when free radicals start outnumbering antioxidants, then there's trouble. Scientists call this *oxidative stress*.

Just exactly how do antioxidants do their work? They appear to perform as described in the next sections.

Vitamin C

Also known as ascorbic acid, vitamin C is a water-soluble nutrient that can be synthesized by many animals, but not by humans. It's an essential nutrient in our diets and functions primarily in the formation of connective tissues such as collagen. Vitamin C is also involved in immunity, wound healing, and allergic responses. As an antioxidant, vitamin C keeps free radicals from destroying the outermost layers of cells.

Vitamin C works with vitamin E. Together they're like two cops on patrol in the body, with vitamin E going undercover to arrest free radicals. It's a ploy that works, since free radicals prefer to latch onto vitamin E rather than to the fatty acids in the cell membrane. Tricked, the free radicals are captured in the raid. Vitamin E is temporarily wounded, but as backup, vitamin C steps in and restores it to its original form.

Evidence exists that links vitamin C to the prevention of cancer. Although most of the results are preliminary, they present very convincing data. In the largest group of studies, vitamin C was significantly protective against stomach cancer. People who ate fewer citrus fruits had a higher incidence of stomach cancer than those without cancer. Similar results have been shown in studies linking vitamin C intake with esophageal cancer, although the results are not as consistent.

So popular is vitamin C that people tend to gobble it by megadoses. Current research shows that taking 250 mg a day provides powerful antioxidant protection. But if you take 500 mg a day, the nutrient can actually promote oxidative stress and block the body's use of other nutrients. Levels over 1,000 mg a day can harm your immune system by interfering with the activity of disease-fighting white blood cells. Too much vitamin C makes the body sop up unhealthy amounts of iron and may interfere with copper absorption.

The best sources of vitamin C in the diet are citrus fruits. Other foods, such as sweet peppers (green and red), collard greens, broccoli, brussels sprouts, cabbage, spinach, potatoes, cantaloupe, kiwifruit, and strawberries, are also excellent sources, providing 30 mg of vitamin C in a serving of less than 50 calories.

Vitamin E

Vitamin E is a fat-soluble vitamin, meaning that it can be stored with fat in the liver and other tissues. Vitamin E is also a component of cells, sandwiched between the fatty layers that make up cell membranes. When free radicals come along, they hitch up to vitamin E, damaging it instead of the rest of the cell membrane. In the process, vitamin E soaks up the free radicals, and the cell is protected from damage.

Acting as a guardian, vitamin E keeps beta-carotene from being destroyed in the body. Of all antioxidant nutrients, vitamin E does the best job of scavenging free radicals.

Vitamin E has gotten a lot of attention for its possible role in preventing heart disease. The stage is set for heart disease when cholesterol builds up in the artery walls, forming plaque and choking off circulation. Vitamin E interrupts this process before it even begins. Without any plaque, your arteries can't get blocked, and you avoid heart disease.

The results of two large research studies lend support to this theory. The two studies, one with women and one with men, found that those people who supplemented with large doses of vitamin E had a lower risk of developing coronary artery disease. The greatest risk reduction was in the men and women who took 100 IU of vitamin E supplements daily.

Unlike other fat-soluble vitamins, vitamin E is not toxic in large doses. There's a possible risk of intestinal problems, however, if you take more than 600 IU a day. Vitamin E is found widely in foods, and the richest sources are vegetable oils and products made from them. Wheat germ and nuts are high in vitamin E, too, and fruits and vegetables supply appreciable amounts.

Beta-Carotene

Beta-carotene is a member of a group of substances known as carotenoids. More than four hundred carotenoids are found in nature, mostly in orange and yellow fruits and vegetables and dark green vegetables. Beta-carotene was the first carotenoid to be isolated and is the most widely studied. Many scientists, however, believe other carotenoids may prove to have more antioxidant power than beta-carotene has. I suspect there's more to come on the carotenoid story.

Once ingested, beta-carotene is converted to vitamin A in the body on an as-needed basis. Beta-carotene's main role as an antioxidant is to detoxify a highly energetic, free-radical-like product called singlet oxygen. Like a server in a cafeteria line, singlet oxygen dishes out its energy to hungry molecules in the line. This process generates many more free radicals. Beta-carotene comes along, shuts the line down by absorbing the singlet oxygen's energy, and puts it out of business. This amazing nutrient can also destroy free radicals after they're formed.

Table 7-3

THE ANTIOXIDANT VITAMINS

	Beta-Carotene	Vitamin C	Vitamin E
Best Sources	Carrots, sweet potatoes, spinach, cantaloupe, broccoli, any dark green leafy vegetables, and orange vegetables and fruits	Citrus fruits and juices, green and red sweet peppers, raw cabbage, berries, kiwifruit, cantaloupe, and green leafy vegetables	Nuts, seeds, raw wheat germ, polyunsaturated vegetable oils, and fish liver oils
Functions	Enhances immune function; complements the antioxidant function of vitamin E	Promotes healthy gums, teeth, and capillaries; maintains normal connective tissue; enhances iron absorption; assists in wound healing	Involved in cellular respiration; assists in the formation of red blood cells; inhibits blood coagulation to prevent blood clots; assists the body in using vitamin K, a fat-soluble vitamin produced in the intestinal tract
Potential Antioxidant Benefits	May reduce the risk of certain cancers, including cancer of the lung, stomach, esophagus, and possibly cancer of the mouth, bladder, colon, and prostate	May block the production of cancer-causing free radicals; has a natural antihistamine effect to counteract cold symptoms and the effects of certain allergens	Appears to reduce exercise-induced lipid peroxidation; may protect against heart disease; may guard tissues against aging; may protect against some cancers
RDA for Adults	No established limits have been set for beta-carotene. A once-a-day vitamin/mineral supplement containing 2,500 IU is safe. You can get that same amount from a large carrot.	60 mg a day—the same amount found in 1 medium-size orange; 100 mg a day for smokers	15 IU a day—the same amount found in 1½ tbsp. of safflower oil. Up to 400 IU a day in supplement form is considered safe by most nutrition experts.
Toxicity	Toxicity is not known because the body carefully controls its conversion to vitamin A. Daily intakes of 20,000 IU of beta-carotene from either food or supplements over several months may cause skin yellowing. This disappears when the dosage is reduced.	The body adapts to high dosages. Dosages higher than 250 mg daily may interfere with immunity. Doses between 5,000 mg and 15,000 mg are known to produce side effects such as burning urination or diarrhea.	Very few cases of vitamin E toxicity have been reported.

Beta-carotene helps ward off diseases by strengthening cell membranes so they can withstand attack. This protective mechanism helps prevent cancer. Beta-carotene also appears to inhibit the growth of cancer cells. Over a decade of research and more than 150 studies have produced evidence that eating fruits and vegetables rich in vitamin C or beta-carotene is linked with a reduced risk of many types of cancer.

The spotlight on beta-carotene and cancer dimmed slightly when the results of a controversial Finnish study were published a few years ago. Researchers studied male smokers who had smoked an average of thirty-five years prior to the study. It appeared that taking beta-carotene was linked to an 18 percent increase in lung cancer among the participants. Naturally, this finding generated a lot of confusion about antioxidant supplementation.

But not to worry. The researchers pointed out that the Finnish diet is high in fat and alcohol and that with their history of smoking, many of the participants may have had cancer before the study got under way. In other words: These results can't be applied to the U.S. population, and certainly not to nonsmokers.

Beta-carotene may prove powerful against heart disease, too. At Harvard, a ten-year health study of male physicians found that men with a history of heart disease who took 50 mg of beta-carotene every other day had half as many heart attacks, strokes, and deaths as those taking placebos. The researchers believe that beta-carotene keeps free radicals from turning bad LDL cholesterol into a form that's even more damaging to the heart. See table 7-3 for a summary of information about the antioxidant vitamins.

Getting Vitamins from Your Diet

In my practice, I ask new clients to fill out a three-day diary of what they eat. I analyze this diary to see where any deficiencies exist. As long as someone's diet is varied with the right mix of carbs, proteins, and fats, there's rarely any need to take vitamin supplements. In some cases, however, I will recommend antioxidant supplementation once a day. For more information on how to supplement with antioxidants, please refer to chapter 9. If you stick to a diet like my Thirty-Day High-Performance Menu Plan found in Appendix A, you can be assured that you're getting an ample supply of vitamins from your food.

CHAPTER 8

Minerals

Major Minerals and Trace Minerals

The body requires minerals in minute amounts. Like vitamins, they don't yield any energy, although some play a behind-the-scenes role in energy production. Unlike vitamins, minerals are indestructible. Neither cooking, food handling, nor processing destroys the mineral content of foods.

There are two categories of minerals: the major minerals and the trace minerals. Major minerals are found in the greatest amounts in the body, and their requirements are higher. Likewise, trace minerals are found in the smallest concentrations and are needed in smaller amounts. Table 8-1 lists the major and minor minerals, with information on their use in exercise. Certain minerals—namely selenium, copper, zinc, and manganese—work as antioxidants. They're listed in table 8-3. The functions of many minerals are still being studied.

Calcium and Iron

Calcium and iron are two hallmarks of good mineral nutrition. If you eat foods naturally high in calcium and iron, you automatically get ample amounts of the major and trace minerals at the same time. That's a tried-and-true maxim of mineral nutrition to keep in mind. So important are these two minerals that they deserve a closer look.

Calcium—The Bone Builder
Of all minerals, calcium has grabbed the most headlines. Why all the attention? Chalk it up to osteoporosis, the bone-thinning disease that strikes older American women in the postmenopausal years. Experts have long felt that bone-building calcium plays a pivotal role in preventing or at least slowing down this crippling illness.

Ninety-nine percent of the calcium in your body is warehoused in your bones and teeth; the other 1 percent resides in blood and soft tissues. The calcium in

Table 8-1

FACTS ABOUT MINERALS

Major Minerals	Exercise-Related Function	Beneficial Effects in Aging	Best Food Sources	Side Effects and Toxicity	RDA for Adults
Calcium	A constituent of body structures; plays a part in muscle growth, muscle contraction, and nerve transmission	Used in the prevention and treatment of osteoporosis	Dairy products and green leafy vegetables	Excessive calcification of some tissues; constipation; mineral absorption problems	800 mg
Phosphorus	Metabolism of carbohydrate, protein, and fat; growth repair and maintenance of cells; energy production; stimulation of muscular contractions	Works with calcium in maintaining healthy bones	Meats, fish, poultry, eggs, whole grains, seeds, and nuts	None known	800 mg
Potassium	Maintenance of normal fluid balance on either side of cell walls; normal growth; stimulation of nerve impulses for muscular contractions; assists in the conversion of glucose to glycogen; synthesis of muscle protein from amino acids	None known	Potatoes, bananas and other fruits, and vegetables	Heart disturbances	1,600–2,000 mg

Sodium	Maintenance of normal fluid balance on either side of cell walls; muscular contraction and nerve transmission; keeps other blood minerals soluble	None known	Found in virtually all foods	Water retention and high blood pressure	500 mg
Chloride	Helps regulate the pressure that causes fluids to flow in and out of cell membranes	Helps keep joints and tendons healthy	Table salt (sodium chloride), kelp, and rye flour	None known	750 mg
Magnesium	Metabolism of carbohydrates and proteins; assists in neuromuscular contractions	Assists in bone growth and in the absorption of other essential minerals; may protect against heart disease	Green vegetables, legumes, whole grains, and seafood	Large amounts are toxic	350 mg for men; 280 mg women

Table 8-1 (continued)

Trace Minerals	Exercise-Related Function	Beneficial Effects in Aging	Best Food Sources	Side Effects and Toxicity	RDA for Adults
Iron	Oxygen transport to cells for energy; formation of oxygen-carrying red blood cells	Required for the production of certain antioxidant enzymes	Liver, oysters, lean meats, and green leafy vegetables	Large amounts are toxic	10 mg for men; 15 mg for women
Iodine	Energy production; growth and development; and metabolism	None known	Iodized salt, seafood, and mushrooms	Thyroid enlargement	150 µg
Chromium	Normal blood sugar and fat metabolism	May assist in cholesterol and blood sugar control	Corn oil, brewer's yeast, whole grains, and meats	Liver and kidney damage	50–200 µg
Fluoride	None known	Bone strengthening	Fluoridated water supplies	Large amounts are toxic	1.5–4.0 mg
Molybdenum	Involved in the metabolism of fats	None known	Milk, beans, breads, and cereals	Diarrhea, anemia, and depressed growth rate	75–250 µg

bones and teeth maintains the structural integrity of these tissues. Without it, we'd probably resemble jellyfish.

Although most of the body's calcium is found in your skeleton, those bones aren't made up of calcium only. They're formed by other nutrients as well. Fluoride, magnesium, copper, zinc, manganese, silicon, and boron help build bone, too. Most of us get fluoride from city water supplies. If you drink well water or purified water that doesn't contain fluoride, ask your physician or dentist whether you should be taking a fluoride supplement. As for the other minerals, eating a varied diet full of seafoods, fruits, vegetables, whole grains, legumes, nuts, and seeds will keep you well supplied.

The calcium in blood and tissue cells helps muscles flex, aids in blood clotting, and moves elements into and out of cells. Any fluctuations in blood and soft tissue calcium can be life-threatening. Fortunately, the body can automatically maintain healthy levels in the blood—as long as you eat plenty of calcium-rich foods. But if a dietary shortage exists, the body withdraws calcium from the storage vaults in the bone and dispatches it to the blood. The greater the draw, the more brittle the bones become. The potential for fractures increases, particularly in the spine, hip, and wrist, and the risk of osteoporosis climbs.

If You're Lactose Intolerant

The team captain of the former Cleveland Browns once broke his foot. He wanted to know what he could do nutritionally to help it heal faster. My initial reaction was: "Not much. Just be sure you're drinking plenty of milk." The calcium in milk would put his injury on the mend. As it turned out, he wasn't a milk drinker due to a problem called *lactose intolerance,* a very common food sensitivity.

People with lactose intolerance lack sufficient lactase, the enzyme required to digest lactose, a sugar in milk that helps you absorb calcium from the intestine. About 70 percent of the world's population is lactose intolerant. The condition causes a range of intestinal disturbances, from gas to severe pain and diarrhea.

If you have lactose intolerance, several options are available to ensure that you get all the calcium you need from milk and milk products. Try drinking small portions of milk (½ cup at a time) at first to see if this amount can be tolerated. Also, aged cheeses and yogurts with active cultures may be more easily digested than straight milk.

New products, such as enzyme-treated Lactaid milk, or Lactaid enzyme tablets for use at home, make milk consumption possible. Another enzyme product, Dairyease, is a tablet that, when taken before meals, assists with lactose digestion and lets you drink milk. I suggested to the Browns captain that he try these products. He did so and had no problems drinking milk from then on.

Partners with Calcium

Calcium is a difficult mineral for your body to absorb, but there are ways to enhance its absorption. Getting plenty of vitamin D is one. Fortunately, vitamin D is the sunshine vitamin, which means that a little time outside on sunny days can help you make enough vitamin D to meet your needs. Also, since milk is the greatest source of calcium in the American diet, vitamin D has been added to milk to enhance calcium absorption.

The protein in milk aids calcium absorption, too. The protein sparks stomach acid secretion, which helps calcium absorption reach peak levels. If you're eating a good nonmilk source of calcium or taking a calcium supplement, it's best to combine it with milk or a meal that contains some protein. This helps boost the amount of calcium your body takes up.

Other Absorption Factors

Have you ever driven down a road, only to be detoured by a roadblock? In a similar fashion, some types of food interact with calcium and block its absorption. Alcohol, for example, decreases calcium absorption and increases calcium losses; people who abuse alcohol tend to have high rates of bone loss.

Eating too much protein may cause your body to lose calcium. It's not clear whether animal and vegetable protein equally affect calcium excretion. Most vegetarians would have trouble consuming enough protein to cause a problem. But if you're taking any kind of protein supplement, check the amount, because it could put you in a calcium deficit.

Other foods can also keep your body from making the most of the calcium you consume. Dietary fibers, oxalic acids, and phytates bind with calcium and keep it from being absorbed in the intestine. Oxalic acid is found in spinach and rhubarb, and phytates are found in wheat bran. If you take a calcium supplement, avoid doing so with high-fiber foods or foods containing these acids.

Megadosing on certain minerals also interferes with calcium absorption. Zinc supplements, for example, can decrease calcium absorption when calcium intake is low. To avoid this, make sure your intake of zinc doesn't go over 100 percent of your RDA for it.

Caffeine causes moderate calcium loss. The amount of caffeine in one cup of coffee (150 mg) can up your calcium needs by 30 to 50 mg each day.

Some drugs can also cause interference. If you use certain antacids, avoid those containing aluminum hydroxide because they increase bone calcium loss and calcium excretion. The antacid Tums, however, is formulated with calcium carbonate, which doesn't block calcium absorption.

Two nondietary risks that affect how your body uses calcium and impair your overall bone health are cigarette smoking and inactivity. Both habits accelerate calcium losses from the body.

Do You Need Calcium Supplements?

The RDA for calcium is based on two things: the amount of calcium in the average American diet and the age we stop building our bones (age twenty-four). From age eleven to twenty-four years, the RDA for men and nonpregnant, nonlactating women is 1,200 mg of calcium per day. The RDA for people older than age twenty-four is 800 mg per day, although this recommendation is controversial.

In 1984 a Consensus Conference on Osteoporosis sponsored by the National Institutes of Health decided to rethink this recommendation for women. It was moved up to 1,200 mg per day before menopause and 1,500 mg after menopause. Officially, the RDA for women age twenty-four and older is still 800 mg, but the medical community now recommends 1,200 mg, and I concur with that recommendation. The RDA for men remains at 800 mg per day. For good health, make sure you're getting the RDA for calcium. This should be easy to do by eating enough calcium-rich foods. Too much calcium in the diet can cause kidney stones in some people.

You'll need to supplement if you can't drink milk or eat milk products. Calcium carbonate and calcium citrate are the two best forms of calcium to take as supplements. Make sure you use a brand from a well-known manufacturer. Obscure supplements are bad news because they're not well regulated. Years ago a group of people got lead poisoning from an off-brand calcium supplement made from cows' bones. After an investigation, it was learned that the cows had been eating grass from a field contaminated with lead from groundwater. No one had bothered to check whether the cows' bones were healthy before being ground up for the supplements. Quality control problems like these are less likely in products made by reputable companies.

Strong Bone R$_X$

Boning up on calcium is critical. Here's a strategy to get the most calcium from your diet and keep your bones healthy:

- Eat a varied, well-balanced diet containing enough calories to meet your energy needs.
- Include three to four servings of milk products every day.
- If you must supplement, take your calcium supplement with milk or a meal to maximize absorption.
- Avoid consuming caffeine and very-high-fiber foods at the same meal with high-calcium foods.
- Don't megadose with other minerals.
- Get plenty of sunshine (for the vitamin D).
- Maintain a regular exercise program. Inactivity is an enemy of calcium. Your body uses this essential mineral better when you're active.
- Don't smoke. Smoking interferes with the body's ability to metabolize and use calcium.
- Keep alcohol consumption to a minimum.

Iron

Just about everybody I know complains about being tired, especially people working full-time jobs and leading active—although hectic—lives. Most of my weary clients have one major question when they walk through my door: "Is it my diet?" It's possible, and low iron could be the offender.

The result of an iron-poor diet is a dragged-out feeling that leaves you with hardly enough get-up-and-go to vacuum the living room or mow the lawn, much less make it through a workout.

One reason I see iron shortages is because so many people are cutting red meat and dark-meat poultry from their diets over concern about fat. But where you find the most iron and other important minerals is in red meat and the dark flesh of poultry and fish. If you're a vegetarian, be sure to consult chapter 23 on good nonmeat sources of iron.

How Iron Works

Iron is the oxygen-carrying particle of the molecules hemoglobin and myoglobin. As part of red blood cells, these molecules transport oxygen from the lungs through the bloodstream to all the cells of your body. Without ample oxygen, your cells can't function efficiently, and they slow down to meet the available oxygen supply. The lower your iron stores dip, the less oxygen that's transported to the cells, and the more tired you'll feel. You'll be fatigued, irritable, and unable to work or exercise at peak levels. You might have headaches and heart palpitations. Biochemically, an absence of iron causes a decrease in the number of red blood cells—a condition called iron-deficiency anemia. Women, take special note: Your iron reserves can be taxed to the limit by blood loss during menstruation.

Potentially, a low-iron diet also signals a zinc deficiency, since both minerals are present in the same foods. A component of more than two hundred enzymes, zinc plays a role in nearly all biologically important functions. Even diets that are marginally deficient in these minerals can cause problems, which often go undetected even through simple blood tests.

With strength training, you're constantly tearing down and rebuilding muscle tissue, creating an enormous demand for blood-building materials like iron. Any type of aerobic exercise that involves pounding of the feet, like jogging, aerobic dancing, and step aerobics, can actually break down red blood cells and potentially cause an iron deficiency, especially when dietary iron is in short supply.

The "Sports Anemia" Myth

You might have heard that athletes can develop something called "sports anemia." Iron levels in the blood of endurance athletes often appear to be low, a deficiency scientists once considered a side effect of training. But now we know otherwise. These athletes don't actually lose iron. Their blood volume increases as a result of training, and this dilutes the amount of iron that's actually measured in the blood. The level of iron is still the same.

Often though, some athletes do succumb to iron deficiencies. But we don't know exactly why. As yet there's no recommendation for increasing iron intake if you're an athlete.

Iron and Heart Disease

A few years ago, there was a lot of hoopla in the press about a study of Finnish men that found a link between heart disease and levels of iron in the blood. The findings bolstered a theory that an excess of iron could lead to heart disease. Little research backed up this theory, however, so no one gave it much credence. In fact, it had been largely discounted for more than a decade—until the results of this Finnish study surfaced.

Eastern Finland has the highest heart attack rates in the world, a health riddle researchers were eager to solve. To get some answers, they studied 1,931 men for five years. What they found was that for each 1 percent increase in the amount of the iron-containing protein ferritin in the blood, heart attack risk increased more than 4 percent.

A second, and very significant, factor was that the men with higher ferritin levels, plus high LDL cholesterol levels, had an even greater risk of heart disease. In other words, high iron and high cholesterol proved to be a double whammy.

This study uncovered a possible explanation for why women have fewer heart attacks than men: Perhaps the lower iron levels in menstruating women protect against heart disease. Until menopause, women have a much lower risk of heart disease compared with men. Scientists used to think that this protective factor was completely due to the control estrogen has over cholesterol levels. Estrogen seems to protect against heart disease until after menopause when levels decline. But maybe that protection is due to low iron stores resulting from menstruation—a factor men don't have.

Conclusions can't be drawn on the basis of only one study. However, the study does raise questions about what should be considered as the normal range of iron in the blood, especially in men. The current RDA for men is 10 mg a day; for women, 15 mg a day.

Fortifying Your Diet with Iron

You can beef up the iron in your diet without adding a lot of beef. Here's how:

✔ Try to keep or add some meat to your diet. See table 8-2 for the "skinniest cuts" of red meat you can enjoy. Lean red meat and the dark meat of chicken and turkey are highest in *heme iron,* the type that comes only from animal

Table 8-2

THE SKINNIEST SIX*		
Cut	**Calories**	**Fat Grams**
Eye of the round	143	4.2
Top round	153	4.2
Top loin	176	8.0
Round tip	157	5.9
Tenderloin	179	8.5
Sirloin	165	6.1

*Per 3-oz. trimmed cooked serving

Source: Data from the Beef Industry Council and Beef Board, 1991.

sources and is best absorbed by the body. A 3- to 4-oz. portion three times a week gives your iron levels a real boost. Another plus is that these meats won't sabotage your efforts at low-fat eating.

✔ Eat fruits, vegetables, and grains that are high in iron. Dietary iron that comes from vegetable sources is called *nonheme iron,* and it's not as well absorbed as that from animal sources. However, if you eat your iron-strong vegetables with meat, you'll absorb more of the iron from the vegetable source. Green leafy vegetables like kale and collards, dried fruits like raisins and apricots, and iron-enriched and fortified breads and cereals are all good plant sources of iron.

✔ Enhance your body's absorption of iron by combining high iron-containing foods with a rich source of vitamin C, which helps the body better absorb iron. Drink some orange juice with your iron-fortified cereal with raisins for breakfast. Or sprinkle some lemon juice on your kale or collards.

✔ Avoid eating very high fiber foods at the same meal with foods high in iron. The fiber inhibits the absorption of iron and many other minerals. The same goes for tea and antacids.

✔ You may need an iron supplement. If you think so, talk to your physician or a registered dietitian. Self-medicating with large doses of iron is risky.

Minerals as Exercise Aids

Some minerals have been touted as exercise aids. A good example is magnesium, a mineral that's in charge of more than four hundred metabolic reactions in the body. One study in particular hints at a link between magnesium and muscle strength. Some men were given 500 mg of magnesium a day, an increase over the RDA of 350 mg. A control group took 250 mg a day, significantly less than the RDA. After both groups trained for eight weeks on weight-training equipment, their leg strength was measured. The supplemented men got stronger, but the control group stayed the same. Researchers aren't yet convinced, however, that magnesium is a strength builder. They caution that the magnesium status of the subjects prior to the study was unknown. That's an important point, since supplementing with any nutrient in which you're deficient is likely to produce some positive changes in performance and health.

Sodium Needs of Exercisers and Athletes

If you exercise vigorously for several hours on a hot and humid day, you can lose up to two quarts of water from sweat each hour, depending on your weight. But water is not the only thing lost in sweat. Along with water go *electrolytes,* minerals that help regulate fluid balance, nerve conduction, and muscle contraction. Sodium, potassium, chloride, and magnesium are all electrolytes that are lost, but sodium is lost in the greatest amounts. The balance between sodium and potassium can be disrupted by excessive sweating. This electrolyte imbalance can lead to painful muscle cramps.

Water lost in sweat must be replaced or your body becomes dehydrated and your exercise performance suffers. But does the sodium lost in sweat need to be replaced as well?

The better trained an athlete you are, the better your body is able to get rid of excess heat and conserve sodium. Becoming used to a hot, humid environment also enhances this ability. And eating a well-balanced diet that contains enough nutrients, including sodium and water, will help you maintain your fluid and electrolyte balance.

With workouts that last less than four hours, you don't need to replace sodium during exercise. If you're a well-trained athlete participating in a standard endurance marathon, for example, you may be sweating up a storm, but you'll reserve enough sodium to complete the competition. Your postevent meal should contain some sodium to replace what you may have lost. But most likely your regular diet contains plenty of sodium to meet your needs.

Sodium and Ultraendurance Events

If you participate in ultraendurance events like triathlons that last longer than four hours, your sodium balance will be affected by the amount you sweat. During such events, even the less-concentrated perspiration of a well-trained athlete depletes sodium to the point that it will need to be replaced *during* the event.

In one study 10 to 20 percent of ultraendurance runners and triathletes and one marathon runner competing in the heat were diagnosed with hyponatremia, which is a depletion of salt in the blood. Symptoms of hyponatremia include drowsiness, muscle weakness and cramping, mental confusion, and seizures.

To replace lost sodium and avoid hyponatremia during long, intense exercise, you can turn to the convenience of fluid-electrolyte drinks. These contain 50 to 100 mg of sodium per cup. I suggest drinking ½ to ¾ cup of a fluid-electrolyte drink every ten to twenty minutes during the event. This amount is enough to replenish your fluid needs if you are an endurance athlete, and your sodium needs if you are an ultraendurance athlete. For more information on fluid-electrolyte drinks, see chapter 16.

The Antioxidant Minerals and Antioxidant Enzymes

Certain minerals are known as antioxidant minerals because they play a protective role against free radical damage. The chief antioxidant minerals are selenium, copper, zinc, and manganese (see table 8.3 for a summary). All are components of enzymes—proteins that bring about chemical changes inside cells.

Table 8-3

THE ANTIOXIDANT MINERALS

	Selenium	Copper	Zinc	Manganese
Best Sources	Cereal bran, whole grain cereals, egg yolk, milk, chicken, seafood, broccoli, garlic, and onions	Whole grain cereals, shellfish, eggs, almonds, green leafy vegetables, and beans	Animal proteins, oysters, mushrooms, whole grain products, and brewer's yeast	Whole grain cereals, egg yolks, dried peas and beans, and green vegetables
Functions	Interacts with vitamin E in normal growth and metabolism	Helps in the formation of hemoglobin and red blood cells by assisting in iron absorption; involved in many enzyme reactions; required for energy metabolism	Needed for the absorption and action of vitamins, particularly the B-complex family; a component of many enzymes involved in metabolism, particularly protein metabolism; works with vitamin C in wound healing	An enzyme activator involved in many metabolic processes, including reproduction and growth
Potential Antioxidant Benefits	Preserves elasticity of the skin; provides possible protection against cancer. Produces glutathione peroxidase, one of the key antioxidant enzymes	Involved with superoxide dismutase (SOD), one of the key antioxidant enzymes	Involved with superoxide dismutase (SOD), one of the key antioxidant enzymes	Involved with superoxide dismutase (SOD), one of the key antioxidant enzymes
RDA for Adults	70 µg for men; 55 µg for women	2 mg	15 mg for men; 12 mg for women	No more than 5 mg a day
Toxicity	Approximately 5 mg a day from food has resulted in hair loss and fingernail changes, according to some research. Higher daily doses have been associated with nausea, abdominal pain, nail and hair changes, diarrhea, fatigue, and irritability.	Toxicity is rare.	Doses higher than 20 mg a day interfere with copper absorption; reduce HDL cholesterol, the beneficial type; and impair the functioning of the immune system.	Large dosages cause vomiting and intestinal problems.

Depending on its role, an enzyme acts like a minister in a marriage ceremony, bonding two parties together, or like a divorce lawyer, splitting them apart, with the enzyme remaining unchanged during the process. Enzymes in the saliva, the stomach, the pancreas, and the small intestine break apart protein, fat, and carbohydrate; other enzymes link or convert one molecule into another, creating new chemical identities for specific functions in the body.

Antioxidant minerals work by supplying the elements your body needs to make antioxidant enzymes. Selenium, for example, produces glutathione peroxidase, an antioxidant enzyme that can turn troublesome free radicals into harmless water.

On its own, selenium has other antioxidant functions. It appears to preserve the elasticity of tissues by delaying the oxidation of fatty acids in proteins. This mineral also works closely with vitamin E in protecting the body against free radicals. Selenium deficiencies have been associated with premature aging. The mineral may also be a safeguard against cancer.

Though technically not an antioxidant mineral, iron is a constituent of the antioxidant catalase, which turns certain types of free radicals into water. Copper, zinc, and manganese work as antioxidants, too. All three help make superoxide dismutase (SOD), an antioxidant enzyme that inactivates certain free radicals. In research with swimmers who consumed copper-rich diets, investigators have seen huge increases in SOD activity as measured by blood tests.

Antioxidant minerals and enzymes form a powerful defense system for the body. That being so, is there a way to pump up these enzymes in your body and fortify yourself even more? Not really. Swallowing extra amounts of minerals in supplement form won't stimulate enzyme activity in your body. Nor will taking enzyme supplements. They're digested just like protein and lose all their enzymatic properties in the process.

Exercise, however, may rev up enzyme activity. In some studies, exercise has been shown to increase the activity of antioxidant enzymes, although results have been inconsistent. Some strong evidence exists showing that when catalase and superoxide dismutase are inhibited, muscles tire out faster. This implies that there may be a relationship between enzymes and muscular exertion. We just don't know for sure.

Getting Minerals from Your Diet

If you choose a variety of foods, all with high nutrient value, you should get the minerals you need to support your fitness needs. Some compelling evidence suggests, however, that supplementation with an antioxidant formula is a good idea for physically active people. I cover this issue fully in chapter 9, so refer to that chapter to see whether you should supplement.

PART THREE

SUPPLEMENTATION FOR ATHLETES AND EXERCISERS

CHAPTER 9

Antioxidant Supplementation

A Case for Antioxidants

Many physically active people think that vitamin and mineral supplements are the elixir for energy and fitness. Since 1972 the sales of dietary supplements have increased sixfold, from $500 million to $3 billion a year. Forty-five percent of all men and 55 percent of women take dietary supplements. On average, those who regularly use nutrient supplements spend $32 a year on vitamin and mineral pills.

I'm repeatedly asked where I stand on taking vitamin and mineral supplements. As I tell my clients, it's far better to consume these nutrients as food. However, enough scientific evidence is piling up to indicate that supplementation with a one-a-day antioxidant formula is a necessity for athletes and other physically active people. Let's look at why.

Preventing Tissue Damage

As explained in chapter 7, exercise produces free radicals that damage body tissues. Does that imply that supplementing with antioxidants can prevent this damage? Perhaps. It appears that antioxidant supplements do play a role in decreasing tissue damage caused by free radicals. Here's why I believe there may be a connection.

Researchers at the Australian Institute of Sport discovered that vitamin E and vitamin C may play an important role in reducing tissue damage in well-trained athletes. In the study, the researchers gave 1,000 IU of vitamin E and 1,000 mg of vitamin C a day or placebos in divided doses at lunch and dinner to three groups of endurance athletes: Olympic cross-country skiers, endurance runners, and triathletes. The supplemented athletes showed about a 25 percent reduction in tissue damage. The researchers also found that antioxidant supplementation also helped the muscles recover and regenerate more quickly following exercise.

Athletes aren't the only ones responding to antioxidant supplementation. In a study of twenty-one sedentary men, researchers at the Antioxidant Research Laboratory at Tufts University gave half the group 800 IU of vitamin E daily for seven weeks. During that time, the subjects participated in an exercise program that involved running downhill on a treadmill for forty-five minutes. The other half took placebos and followed the same seven-week exercise program. Half of the men in each group were in their twenties; the other half ranged in age from fifty-five to seventy-four years old.

All the vitamin E–supplemented men excreted in their urine far less of a by-product that indicates tissue breakdown. Plus, blood tests showed significantly reduced levels of chemicals that promote inflammation. These findings led the researchers to conclude that vitamin E may help prevent muscle damage and reduce muscle soreness.

Preventing oxidative stress—a condition where free radicals outnumber antioxidants—may be as simple as supplementing with an antioxidant, according to a study from the Washington University School of Medicine in St. Louis. For one month, unexercised medical students took high doses of antioxidants daily: 1,000 IU of vitamin E, 1,250 mg of vitamin C, and 37.5 mg of beta-carotene. The doses were divided into five capsules a day. Part of the group took placebos.

Prior to supplementation, the students ran at a moderate pace on a treadmill for about forty minutes, followed by five minutes of high-intensity running to exhaustion. The same exercise bout was repeated after supplementation.

The researchers observed that oxidative stress caused by exercise was high prior to supplementation. In other words, a lot of tissue damage was going on. With antioxidants, some oxidative stress was still caused by exercise, but it wasn't as great. The researchers concluded that taking antioxidants offered protection against tissue damage.

Antioxidant Supplements and Performance

If you take antioxidants, will you be able to bike farther, work out longer, or get across the finish line faster? Whether antioxidant supplementation really improves performance hasn't been adequately answered by research. We do know that if you're undernourished—that is, you have a vitamin deficiency—you'll definitely feel better and perform better by correcting that deficiency. But if your diet is already high in antioxidants, supplementing it with extra antioxidants may not make much of a difference in your performance.

Antioxidants for Strength Trainers and Cross Trainers

Most of the research in antioxidant supplementation has been done with endurance athletes. But what about people who cross-train with aerobics and strength training? If you work out consistently, you're tearing down a lot of tissue. Not only that, muscles generate free radicals during and after exercise. For these reasons, I feel that there may be some correlation. That being the case, you may want to take some extra measures to protect yourself from the potential onslaught of free radicals.

In most of the people I've worked with, I've seen dietary deficiencies in vitamin E. One of the reasons is that active, health-conscious people typically go on diets that are low in fat, and dietary fat is one of the best sources of vitamin E. What's more, some active people, particularly strength trainers, are known to limit their intake of fruit. Misinformed, they think the fructose it contains will turn up as body fat on their physiques. But by cutting out fruits, they cut out foods that are loaded with the antioxidants beta-carotene and vitamin C.

Supplementing with Antioxidants

For physically active people, I recommend once-a-day supplementation with a multivitamin/mineral tablet containing antioxidant nutrients. If you work out more than four times a week, are not eating at least two servings a day of antioxidant-rich foods, or are older than age sixty-five, then you're definitely a candidate for supplementation.

At this point, the exact antioxidant requirement has not been nailed down. Rather than wait for the final word on it, I feel that moderate use of antioxidant supplements may be beneficial. Based on available evidence on antioxidants, I suggest the following daily intakes:

- 10,000 to 20,000 IU of beta-carotene
- 100 to 400 IU of vitamin E
- 200 to 300 mg of vitamin C
- Up to 50 micrograms (μg) of selenium

The best sources of these nutrients are food, because they provide health-giving phytochemicals and combinations of antioxidants like vitamin C, vitamin E, and beta-carotene, which are clearly interactive when it comes to fighting free radicals. Admittedly, it's difficult to get all the antioxidants you need from food. According to Pat O. Daily, M.D., and Patti Tveit Milligan, M.S., R.D., writing in *IDEA Today*, here's what you'd have to eat in one day to fulfill your antioxidant requirement:

- 1 apple
- 2–3 dried apricots
- 1 banana
- 1 orange
- 2 tablespoons of almonds

- 5 to 6 oysters
- 1 cup brown rice
- ½ cup broccoli
- 1 tablespoon of molasses
- 1 cup spinach or kale
- 1 cup wheat germ
- 1 cup black beans
- 1 cup wheat germ
- ½ cup brussels sprouts
- 1 cup sunflower seeds
- 1 medium sweet potato

That's a pretty hefty volume of food to swallow! Current guidelines from the American Dietetic Association tell us to eat three or more servings a day of vegetables and two or more servings of fruit. Unfortunately, only 9 percent of all Americans eat these recommended amounts, according to estimates. That's further justification for supplementing—but only if you have an antioxidant-rich diet already in place. A poor diet with supplements is still a poor diet.

I suggest that you eat at least five servings of vegetables and four servings of fruits every day, as the High-Performance Menus in Appendix A provide. Include a variety of green, orange, yellow, and citrus fruits in your diet. Although you should eat nuts, seeds, and oils sparingly, have some of them every day to ensure an optimum intake of vitamin E. Toasted wheat germ is also a flavorful way to add some E to your diet.

As for supplements, any commercial one-a-day-type multivitamin/mineral tablet with an antioxidant formula of vitamin C, vitamin E, and beta-carotene, as well as the antioxidant minerals, will give you the extra protection you need to keep your performance levels high.

CHAPTER 10

Creatine—The Antidote to Low Energy

What Is Creatine?

More power and less fatigue—that's what being active is all about. But some days, it's all you can do to drag yourself out of bed, let alone to the gym or exercise class for a workout.

Could it be you're having an energy crisis?

One problem might be nutrition. Good nutrition is absolutely essential for energy. You're not going to perform if you've skipped some meals or cut your calories to drastically low levels. But suppose you're doing everything right, and you still need some extra oomph. What's the solution?

It's creatine, a nonvitamin nutrient manufactured naturally in the body and available in some foods. Not since carbohydrate loading was introduced thirty years ago has there been a bona fide nutritional energy-extender for active people. But even carbohydrate loading was really only for endurance athletes competing in long-distance events like marathons and triathlons. There wasn't anything for regular exercisers who strength-train or engage in other types of short-burst, high-intensity exercise. Creatine may be the best-kept secret in exercise and nutrition today.

The Magic of Creatine

The discovery of creatine reads like a good mystery novel. In 1984 Dr. Roger Harris, a physiologist at the Animal Health Trust in Newmarket, England, tried giving a dose of creatine to a horse as part of a research experiment. But when the animal balked, Dr. Harris got the creatine dose instead of the horse. Soon afterward he found that his blood concentration of creatine had shot sky-high.

This event gave scientists the first clue that creatine could pass through the stomach undigested and travel straight to the bloodstream. Next came the realization that creatine could be taken up by the muscles, much like glycogen is during carbohydrate loading. Glycogen is the fuel that powers muscles during exercise. Muscles can load up with extra glycogen after we load up on dietary carbohydrate. And now it appears that muscles can do the same with creatine.

Scandinavian researcher Eric Hultman, Ph.D., known as "the father of carbo loading," is one of the principal scientists who discovered that creatine supplements can boost performance. The sports scientists now doing this cutting-edge research say creatine is the biggest thing since the discovery of carbohydrate loading.

How Creatine Works

Creatine is produced in the liver and kidneys—about 2 g a day—from arginine, glycine, and methionine, three nonessential amino acids. It's carried by the blood, to be stored in the muscles, heart, and other body cells. About 95 percent of the body's creatine heads to the muscles. Inside muscle cells, it's turned into a compound called creatine phosphate (CP). Creatine phosphate serves as a tiny energy supply, enough for several seconds of action. That's why CP works best over the short haul, in activities that require short, fast bursts of activity. Creatine phosphate also replenishes your cellular reserves of ATP, the molecular fuel that provides the power for muscular contractions. With more ATP around, you can do more work.

Available as a supplement, creatine holds great promise if you lift weights, cycle, row, swim, sprint, or play sports like soccer and ice hockey. Its potential for extending energy in these types of activity seems tremendous. And unlike most nutritional supplements, it seems to live up to its energy-producing claims. Consider the following information.

In one study, eight physical education students took creatine supplements for five days while another group took placebos. Following the supplementation period, the students exercised on a cycle ergometer, performing 130 pedal revolutions for 10 seconds, interspersed with 30 seconds of rest. The next day they upped their revolutions to 140 to induce greater fatigue.

Compared with the placebo group, the creatine group could do more revolutions per minute over the final moments of each exercise bout. The placebo group tired out much sooner than the creatine group. Creatine supplementation maximized energy for this type of short-duration activity and postponed fatigue.

The exciting discovery that you can load creatine into your muscles like you load glycogen is a real breakthrough. Instead of quickly tiring near the end of any short-burst, high-intensity activity, you can keep going. The extra creatine boosts the pace of energy production in the muscle cell and allows the muscle fibers to work harder for longer.

A Real-Life Success Story

Intrigued by creatine's potential, I began to use it with some of my clients—and with good results. One of these clients was Matt, a seventeen-year-old swimmer with Olympic aspirations who competed in the 200- and 100-meter breaststrokes, both power events. My first task was to get his nutrition up to par. At 6 ft. 2 and 154 lb., he was really a beanpole, with little muscle to power him for his sport.

Like a lot of busy people, Matt had a full load—school, homework, and training—but wasn't eating enough nutrients and calories to give him much energy. I created a diet for him consisting of 3,500 daily calories in food and 1,000 daily calories in liquid supplements. Over a month's time, he gradually added the liquid supplements to the diet to get him up to the 4,500-calorie mark. Within four months, he had gained a badly needed 10 lb., and at least 60 percent of that weight was pure muscle.

Still, Matt was looking for something else to enhance his performance. So we tried creatine, using a research-tested dosage schedule. He took 20 g of creatine for five days. This dosage has been found to boost creatine content in the muscles by up to 25 percent. In training, he felt the benefits immediately. The reason for his dramatic response, I feel, was that his creatine stores were low prior to supplementation because he had been eating poorly for so long. Creatine supplementation gave him the jump start he needed. By successfully combining good nutrition with creatine supplementation, Matt went on to win his state events.

Creatine Cuts Muscle Burn

Creatine supplementation also cuts lactic acid levels in the blood. Lactic acid buildup is what makes your muscles "burn" after repeated contractions. It's a waste product of short-burst exercise that accumulates in the muscles and blood. Lots of lactic acid in the muscles wears you down while you're working out.

Lactic acid buildup is still a major cause of fatigue, but so is creatine depletion. The results of research into creatine prove this point. In one study, researchers looked at creatine levels in sprinters and found that their muscle supply fell markedly according to the length of the sprints. After 100 meters, creatine levels dropped by 50 percent; after 200 meters, 59 percent; and after 400 meters, 90 percent. When creatine stores were fully emptied, complete fatigue set in.

Less Muscle Soreness

If all this news isn't enough, creatine phosphate (the form that works inside cells) also neutralizes the free radicals produced by intense exercise, thereby decreasing the amount of muscle tissue damage that causes soreness. So each time you exercise hard, you can return to training sooner due to less muscle soreness. All this results in a great performance-enhancing aid—one that's safe, legal, and really works.

A Side Effect of Creatine

A known side effect of taking creatine is that it can increase body weight. In a study of eighteen runners, half the runners were given creatine for six days, and nine were given a placebo. They ran a hilly six-mile course before and after supplementation. The placebo group performed best. They either maintained or improved their times, whereas the creatine group ran more slowly. Interestingly, the creatine runners gained an average of 1 lb. in weight. According to the researchers, it's the weight gain that may have slowed them down.

Could the weight gain have been muscle? If so, does this mean creatine helps you develop muscle? There's no proof that creatine supplementation changes body composition. In fact, some researchers say the gain is water weight. But if creatine gives you the energy to exercise more intensely, that effort could translate into less body fat, more lean muscle, and greater strength.

Getting Creatine into Your Muscles

Creatine supplements swell the ranks of creatine in your muscles. This gives the working muscles another fuel source, in addition to glycogen from carbohydrates. The question is, how much creatine do you need? The average daily intake from food is about 1 g.

About 120 to 184 g of creatine are stored in muscle. Whether you're on the low end or high end of that scale may depend on your diet. If you eat meat, you've got creatine in your diet. Not eating meat doesn't mean that you're creatine-deficient, since the body manufactures its own. But some of the research indicates that vegetarians might fall into the lower end of the range.

Although you wouldn't want to, you can get creatine from raw meat and fish. When these foods are cooked, however, their creatine content falls, so it's hard to obtain the amount you'd want to supplement. To match what's recommended to enhance performance, you'd have to scarf down about 4 lb. of steak a day! That's certainly not the kind of food plan that meets a low-fat diet guideline. And even if you chowed down on other sources—fish, oysters, prunes, mushrooms, brewer's yeast, nuts, beer, asparagus, and wine—you'd fall short of recommended levels.

Creatine Supplements

Since it's difficult to get from food the amount of creatine you need to enhance performance, supplements are available at health food stores nationwide. Peter

Greenhaff, one of the world's leading creatine researchers, recommends 5 g (usually a teaspoon, but check the label) dissolved in warm water and taken four times a day for five days to load your muscles. Any more than that may just go to waste, as the body simply can't use it. From there, he says, 2 g a day—about half a teaspoon—will keep levels sufficiently high. Keep in mind that high doses, more than 2 g a day, can lead to weight gain. What's more, there have been reports about possible liver and kidney damage from taking daily dosages of 40 g or more. Check with your physician before supplementing with creatine.

With all the fanfare, creatine supplements are beginning to be seen on the shelves in health food stores. There are reports that all of the supplements are not pure creatine but may be cut with fillers. Likely due to the fillers, many products suggest higher doses than if the products were pure. Prices vary greatly among products.

Very few experts are downplaying the effectiveness of creatine supplementation. Dr. Robert Maughan, an exercise physiologist at the University of Aberdeen in Scotland, has been an outspoken critic of creatine. But now even he concedes that "there's now little doubt that creatine can improve performance."

Admittedly, creatine supplementation is still in its infancy. But who knows? It may soon become an accepted nutritional practice for anyone who wants to reach his or her level of high performance.

CHAPTER 11

My Firming Formula

A Supplement for Strength Trainers and Cross Trainers

What if a formula existed that would make you feel stronger and more energetic, plus help you build a fit, firm body? Wouldn't you want to use it in your nutrition and exercise program? Of course!

There is such a formula—one that helps retool your body composition for more lean muscle and less fat, elevates energy levels, and does it naturally, as long as you're following a consistent strength-training program.

The formula is 11 oz. of carbohydrates and protein in liquid form taken immediately following your strength-training routine. This is the time your body is best able to use these nutrients for muscle firming and fat burning. The supplement I use with my clients is a Gatorade product, GatorPro. Convenient to take to the gym for a quick refresher after your workout, GatorPro provides 360 calories, 59 g of carbohydrate, 17 g of protein, and 7 g of fat. Be sure to drink it cold. Other products with similar nutrient profiles should also be effective.

If you'd rather drink your carb-protein supplement at home, try my homemade meal replacer. Simply mix a packet of Carnation Instant Breakfast with 8 oz. skim milk, 1 banana, and 1 tablespoon of peanut butter, and blend until smooth. One serving gives you 438 calories, 70 g of carbohydrate, 17 g of protein, and 10 g of fat.

Early on I used this formula or GatorPro with some of my bodybuilding clients and soon started observing some major differences in their muscle growth patterns. Then I thought: Why not use it on regular exercisers? I did, and it resulted in some remarkable gains for those who used it. Stephen D. is a good example.

A Case Study

At 6 ft. 10, Stephen weighed 265 lb. at 23 percent body fat—somewhat on the high side. His goal was to alter his body composition so that less of his weight was fat and more was muscle. At the time I began to work with him, he was eating only 3,000 calories a day, far too low for his height. No wonder he had such a high percentage of body fat. His metabolism had slowed down, and he was storing more fat than he was burning. He was also low on energy. Right away I upped his calories to 4,850. For exercise, he started a program of aerobics and strength training.

Stephen began eating a lot of food, including 23 bread servings, 10 fruits, 10 vegetables, and 2 milks. But don't forget: A tall man can handle plenty of food. A portion of his calories came from a single serving of GatorPro, a meal replacer containing carbs, protein, and other nutrients. As I instructed him to, Stephen drank GatorPro immediately after his workout.

Before long he was bursting at the seams—literally. His shirts were getting tight around his shoulders and upper arms, but his waist size had stayed nice and trim. All this proved one thing: His fat-to-muscle ratio had changed dramatically. Body fat was down, muscle weight was up. Just what he had hoped for.

Today Stephen's body-fat percentage is 10.7, down significantly from 23 percent. He weighs a fit and toned 229. Not only that, he's now a college student, a personal trainer, an aerobics teacher, and a bike shop employee. Full of energy, he's performing well mentally and physically and plans to continue this nutrition program. It's definitely become a lifestyle for him.

I've had many similar cases in which people changed their nutrition program, started strength training, and used a carb-protein supplement right after exercise. Each time, the common denominator has been a stronger, firmer body, plus loads of energy.

Why This Formula Works

So what's going on here? Why does this formula help muscles get stronger and firmer? Exercise, of course, is the stimulus. You challenge your muscles by working out, and they respond by shaping up. But they need protein and carbs *in combination* to create the right environment for muscle growth.

Protein and carbohydrates stimulate the release of certain hormones in your body. The two most important are insulin and growth hormone. Insulin is a powerful factor in building muscle. It enhances the transport of amino acids into cells, reassembles amino acids into body tissue, and prevents muscle wasting and tissue loss.

Growth hormone increases the rate of protein production by the body, spurring on muscle-building activity. It also promotes fat burning. Both hormones are directly involved in muscle development.

In recent years exercise scientists have started experimenting with exercisers and athletes to see what effect, if any, carb-protein supplements could have on hormones. Here's the latest work showing why science supports my firming formula:

✔ In one study, fourteen normal-weight men and women were fed test meals containing various amounts of protein (in grams): 0 (a protein-free meal), 15.8, 21.5, 33.6, and 49.9, along with 58 g of carbohydrate. Blood samples were taken at intervals following the meal. The protein-containing meals produced the greatest rise in insulin, compared with the protein-free meal. This study points out that protein clearly has an insulin-enhancing effect.

✔ At the University of Texas in Austin, nine experienced male strength trainers were given either water (which served as the control), a carbohydrate supplement, a protein supplement, or a carbohydrate/protein supplement. They took their designated supplement immediately after working out and again two hours later. Right after exercise and throughout the next eight hours, the researchers drew blood samples to determine the levels of various hormones in the blood, including insulin, testosterone (a male hormone also involved in muscle growth), and growth hormone.

The most significant finding was that the carbohydrate/protein supplement triggered the greatest elevations in insulin and growth hormone. Clearly, the protein works hand in hand with postexercise carbs to create a hormonal environment that's highly conducive to muscle growth.

Muscle Energy

My clients who use the firming formula report higher energy levels. That's because supplementing with a carb-protein mixture replenishes glycogen, which translates into more energy for strength training. The harder you can work out, the better your muscular development.

Drinking protein and carbs after a workout actually speeds up the body's glycogen-making process, better than just carbs alone. In one study, nine men cycled for two full hours during three different sessions to deplete their muscle glycogen stores. Immediately after each exercise bout and again two hours later, the men drank either a straight carb supplement, a straight protein supplement, or a carbohydrate/protein supplement. By looking at actual biopsies of the muscles, the researchers observed that the rate of muscle glycogen storage was significantly faster when the carb/protein mixture was consumed.

Why such speed? It's well known that eating carbs after prolonged endurance helps restore muscle glycogen. When protein is consumed along with carbs, there's a surge in insulin. Biochemically, insulin is like an acceleration pedal. It races the body's glycogen-making motor—in two ways. First, it speeds up the movement of glucose and amino acids into cells, and, second, it activates a special enzyme crucial to glycogen synthesis.

Supplementing during Exercise

In 1993 a group of scientists at California State University–Chico added a new twist to the research: What would happen if you sipped a carb-protein supplement *while* working out? Typically, when you exercise, insulin tends to drop off—not the situation you want when you're trying to develop muscle. The scientists reasoned that during strength training, it would be beneficial to have elevated blood glucose, which leads to higher levels of insulin. Possibly, this increased insulin could stimulate the body's protein-making machinery.

To test the scientists' theory, ten bodybuilders were signed up for the experiment. They were given either a liquid meal consisting of 13 g of protein, 31.9 g of carbohydrate, and 2.6 g of fat or a placebo that was devoid of any nutrients.

The subjects drank this meal thirty minutes before a two-hour strength-training session and at fifteen-minute intervals during exercise. They also drank it before and intermittently during two hours of rest. Blood samples were drawn at various times during the experiments and tested in a lab.

The results showed that intermittent feeding of a carb-protein supplement during strength training kept blood glucose at or above normal levels. The feeding also significantly increased insulin levels. The scientists concluded that this reaction could possibly speed up muscle growth.

The Role of Diet

Building fit, firm muscle—is it as easy as just exercising and drinking a carb-protein concoction during and after your workout? No, there's a lot more to it than that. You can't neglect a good diet—like my high-performance nutrition program mapped out for you in Appendix A.

You've got to eat enough quality calories each day to fuel your body for exercise and activity. If you don't get in enough calories, you're going to upset this hormonal climate that's so important to getting fit, not to mention that you won't have much energy to exercise. Research shows that low-calorie dieting makes growth hormone levels nose-dive, so the hormone can't exert its fat-burning or muscle-building effect.

The point is, you need to stay on a diet that provides adequate energy so that your hormonal climate stays right and you're well energized for exercise. Then take my firming formula right after your workouts to literally jump-start your muscle-developing machinery.

PART FOUR

CONTROVERSIAL SUPPLEMENTS

CHAPTER 12

The Truth about Some Supplements

False Promises

Confused by all the nutritional supplement ads you see in health and fitness magazines? No wonder. Claims like "Lose weight while you sleep," "Muscle growth stimulator," or "Reduce fatigue" can be enticing. You're led to believe you can become strong just by taking a pill or a powder.

Some words of warning, however. A lot of these claims are based on meager and unreliable research. And that spells trouble. When a supplement sounds too much like a drug, the Food and Drug Administration (FDA) gets into the act. In 1991 the FDA cracked down on the distributors of a popular, widely sold supplement powder. The product in question was formulated with thirty substances, including amino acids, minerals, and herbs, and billed in ads as a steroid alternative. The FDA felt that this advertising was misleading, intended to make the product sound like a muscle-building drug. In response to the FDA, the company changed some of its claims. Despite the FDA's vigilance, many supplement companies still make claims in fitness magazines that their products "build muscle fast."

But don't bet on it. To date, no dietary supplement has been proven to build muscle, burn fat, or perform any such body-shaping miracles.

Possible Side Effects

Did you know you could actually get sick from some of these products? The side effects of many supplements already have been reported to the FDA. And some of them aren't too pleasant, like stomach pain, nausea, dizziness, vomiting, diarrhea, and cardiovascular problems. What's not clear are the causes. One theory holds that these supplements often contain mystery ingredients, which react adversely in combination with each other.

Some mail-order supplements can be just as mysterious. Often you just don't know what's in them. And if you do, you can't be sure the supplement really contains what it says it does.

Case in point: Not long ago, I worked with an eighteen-year-old marathoner, an Olympic contender, who was diagnosed as anemic. Even though he had been strength-training for four years, he was still a "string bean." What's more, his performance had slipped.

This athlete had stopped taking the iron supplement prescribed by his doctor. Instead, he was using some mail-order supplements. I asked him to bring all of them to my office so I could analyze his diet. What I found was a very expensive batch of supplements: protein enzymes, a vitamin/mineral supplement that contained some iron, kelp tablets (kelp contains iron, but the body doesn't use it very well), a carbohydrate supplement, and a vitamin E supplement.

A red flag went up immediately. None of the labels told me exactly what was in the supplements. I was concerned for three reasons. First, my client wasn't getting what he needed nutritionally. To make matters worse, his diet was too low in calories. Second, supplements from off-brand manufacturers can be toxic, especially if ingredients like kelp were harvested under environmentally poor conditions. Third, he was wasting his money.

Time for a new strategy. For starters, I suggested that he resume taking his prescription iron supplement. Next I recommended an antioxidant vitamin/mineral formula and a separate vitamin E supplement, both from a recognized, well-established pharmaceutical company. He also needed to fortify his diet with iron-rich foods like lean red meat, as well as with high vitamin C foods like fruits and vegetables. Vitamin C would help his body better absorb the iron he so desperately needed. Along with that, I advised him to increase his calories from food to better fuel his training.

He stuck to the strategy. At the end of four months, he had resolved his iron deficiency and improved his competitive performance. He now has his sights set on the next Olympics.

Questionable Supplements

Once a shred of evidence surfaces that a certain nutrient may improve health or performance, the next place you see that nutrient is in a new supplement product. Many supplement manufacturers distort nutritional research findings, using this information to give their products an aura of credibility and authority. This practice is nothing short of quackery, since consumers are tricked into buying something they don't really need. What follows is a description of twenty-three substances I feel have been deceptively marketed to fitness-conscious consumers. Many of their advertised uses are questionable, controversial—and definitely unproven. Here's a rundown.

Amino Acid Supplements

Amino acid supplements are heavily marketed to bodybuilders and other strength-training athletes with claims that they build muscle as a safe alternative to steroid drugs. But these supplements are bought not only by bodybuilders but also by average exercisers lured by promises that amino acids, the building blocks of protein, build lean mass and burn fat. The historical marketing angle for amino acids is that they are nitrogen-containing compounds, and their use is believed to cause nitrogen retention in the body. Supposedly, nitrogen retention initiates protein formation at the cellular level and, ultimately, muscle growth.

The more recent excitement over amino acids comes from research showing that certain amino acids, injected into the bloodstream in large amounts, trigger the release of growth hormone, a protein substance that promotes fat mobilization and makes cells multiply faster. But those who buy amino acid preparations don't take injections of amino acids; they take oral supplements. In most cases, it's too difficult to take a high-enough oral dose to even affect growth hormone secretion.

One well-publicized study, however, did demonstrate that an oral dose of two amino acids (1,200 mg of arginine and 1,200 mg of lysine) taken on an empty stomach stimulated growth hormone secretion. But that was all. There were no muscular gains.

Studies on amino acids and muscle building are continuing, but at this time, supplementing with amino acids has no proven benefit. When you take amino acids, you're really taking extra protein. If not used right away, the surplus can be packed away as fat. What's more, too much protein can overload the kidneys and possibly lead to kidney damage. The long-term effects of amino acid supplementation are unknown.

Not long ago I read the results of a study in which amino acid supplement products taken from a health food store were analyzed for their content. Most of them contained the amino acid glycine as their *primary* constituent, regardless of what was stated on the label. Glycine is a relatively inexpensive amino acid—which explains why some unscrupulous supplement manufacturers would use it. If you purchase amino acid supplements, you could be getting ripped off.

The next time you're tempted to take amino acids, consider this: A mere one ounce of chicken contains 7,000 mg of amino acids—the equivalent of an entire bottle of amino acids. And for that you'd pay about $10!

L-Tryptophan Users Beware

Tryptophan is an amino acid supplement once used by athletes to increase strength and muscle mass, although it does neither. Other people have used tryptophan to relieve insomnia, depression, anxiety, and premenstrual tension. In 1989, thousands of Americans developed a crippling illness called eosinophilia-myalgia syndrome after taking tainted tryptophan made by a Japanese chemical company. Although some recovered rapidly after stopping the supplements, thirty-one people died.

Others had lingering damage, including inflammation, muscle pain and fatigue, scarring of connective tissue around muscle, and deterioration of nerves and muscle. Unfortunately, there aren't many effective treatments for this syndrome, particularly in its later stages, and many victims become permanently disabled.

As a result of this scare, tryptophan was yanked from the market. I think this sad story underscores one of the biggest problems with supplements today: As a consumer, you can't distinguish between a contaminated product and a pure one, because no regulation, product testing, or quality control are applied to these products.

Enzymes

Products such as papain, derived from papaya, or bromelain from pineapple are sold in pill form as enzymes purporting to help your body digest protein. But remember: Enzymes are protein, and your body digests them like a piece of chicken or fish. What's more, your body has its own special enzyme (pepsin) that initiates the breakdown of protein. It doesn't need outside help. So buyer beware. All the talk about taking enzymes to help your body digest protein is gibberish.

Carnitine

Discovered in 1905, this proteinlike substance was once thought to be a vitamin and was even named vitamin B_T. Now scientists know carnitine is not an essential nutrient, since the liver and kidneys can synthesize it without any help from food. Carnitine is found in red meat and other animal products, and most people consume between 50 mg and 300 mg of this nutrient a day. Even if you don't eat that much, your body can produce its own from the amino acids lysine and methionine. About 98 percent of the body's carnitine is stored in the muscles.

Carnitine deficiencies are rare yet serious. Muscles can weaken, fats can build up in muscle fibers, and eventually a coma or heart attack could occur. Deficiencies have been seen in vegetarians who eat no animal products.

Carnitine's main job in the body is to transport fatty acids into cells to be burned as energy. Because of this role, many claims have been attached to carnitine; for example, can supplementing with it lend a hand in burning fat? Some investigators feel the demand for carnitine is increased during exercise because it's mobilized by the body to burn fat as fuel for the activity. But this notion has been challenged.

In a study at Case Western Reserve University, researchers administered carnitine intravenously to subjects (others were given placebos) just before they began exercising on a cycle ergometer. The researchers then monitored the effect of supplementation on carnitine levels in the muscles. But no increase was observed. They also checked to see whether the supplement influenced the use of stored fat and carbohydrate during workouts. The result: No effect whatsoever.

Still other researchers have tried to find a connection between taking carnitine and extending endurance. A few studies have suggested that supplementing with 2 g of carnitine a day for a month improves oxygen use during exercise. The results of most studies are contradictory, however. Some studies find a benefit; others don't.

These findings tell me there's still much to be learned about carnitine's role in physical performance. Carnitine is being used experimentally in other areas, including the treatment of heart disease and in kidney dialysis therapy. But unless you're under a physician's supervision, I don't recommend carnitine supplementation because we know so little about its real effect on the body.

Boron

This essential trace mineral has been advertised as a muscle builder, although there's no proof for the claim. Some early research showed that it promoted growth in animals with dietary deficiencies. But using that research to say boron helps develop muscle in humans is making quite a leap of faith.

One positive finding about boron is its role in mineral metabolism. It helps the body properly use other minerals, guards against calcium losses, and thus may be a factor in preventing osteoporosis. The richest sources of boron in the diet are found in foods like soy meal, prunes, raisins, peanuts, and hazelnuts. Since so little is needed, however, you really don't need supplemental boron.

Chromium

Flip through any health and fitness magazine today and you're bound to find an ad for chromium, a nutrient that's been billed as a fat burner and a muscle builder. In fact, it's the most-hyped mineral today. Valid scientific evidence just doesn't support these claims, however.

Chromium is an essential trace mineral that helps the body turn carbohydrates and fats into energy. It increases the effectiveness of insulin by helping transport glucose into cells for energy. Chromium is also involved in the synthesis of protein. Dietary sources include brewer's yeast, whole grain cereals, meats, raw oysters, mushrooms, apples with skins, wine, and beer. The body absorbs only about 3 percent of dietary chromium.

Virtually all of this chromium is lost in the urine. Two factors can speed up this loss: eating simple sugars and exercising. Many active people stick to—and rightly so—a high-carbohydrate diet. Sometimes though, these diets are too high in juices or processed foods, both sources of hidden simple sugars. A diet overloaded with simple sugars can force chromium from the body.

Exercise has been shown in research to do the same. One study in particular measured the chromium losses of nine runners and found that their losses were twice as great on exercise days as on nonexercise days. Conceivably, anyone in a chromium-deficient state could have problems metabolizing carbohydrates and fats, jeopardizing energy levels and performance.

If an active lifestyle affects chromium status, could supplementation give your body the chromium it needs to metabolize needed nutrients? Let's take a closer look at the evidence.

Most supplemental chromium is sold as chromium picolinate. One of its most alluring claims is that it helps build muscle mass. The research results on this issue are confusing at best. Some studies show that it does, others show it doesn't, and still others show no change. Most of the studies to date have been very poorly designed and have used inaccurate methods of measuring body composition.

The best and most comprehensive study I've seen was conducted at the University of Massachusetts a few years ago. Thirty-six football players were given either a placebo or 200 μg of chromium picolinate daily for nine weeks during spring training, a period in which they worked out with weights and engaged in a running program. Before, during, and after supplementation, the researchers assessed the players' diets, urinary chromium losses, girth of various body parts, percentages of body fat and muscle, and strength. Percentages of body fat and muscle were measured by underwater weighing, one of the most precise methods to gauge body composition. The findings: Chromium supplementation *did not* help build muscle, enhance strength, or burn fat.

These findings are supported by one of the leading research centers in the United States—the USDA Human Nutrition Research Center in Grand Forks, North Dakota, where chromium picolinate was first synthesized. Researchers there have studied chromium extensively and agree that it has no effect on strength or body composition.

Some words of warning about chromium supplementation: Chromium picolinate is a mixture of chromium and picolinic acid, a substance that is reported to help the body better absorb chromium. Picolinic acid, however, has been reported to alter the shape of cells and interfere with their inner workings. Furthermore, it causes the body to excrete other trace minerals and alters the metabolism of iron. Like two passengers trying to hop on the same taxi, chromium competes with iron at a critical site in the hemoglobin-making process. Given these drawbacks and the fact that chromium picolinate doesn't live up to its claims, supplementation is nutritional bungee-jumping at best.

Vanadium

This trace mineral is found in vegetables and fish. The body needs very little vanadium, and more than 90 percent of it is excreted in the urine. As a supplement, vanadium is supposed to have a tissue-building effect by moving glucose into the muscles faster and elevating insulin to promote growth. I hate to keep pouring cold water on the latest "nutritional breakthrough," but there's no truth to this tale, either.

Experts at the USDA Human Nutrition Research Center in Grand Forks, North Dakota, where the most authoritative work on vanadium has been conducted, say there's no reason for anyone to supplement with this mineral, even people who have trouble metabolizing glucose. At high doses, vanadium is extremely toxic. Avoid this supplement at all costs.

Phosphate

For a long time, athletes have experimented with phosphate loading as a way to extend performance. Phosphate is a type of salt made from phosphorus, the second most abundant mineral in the body. The supplement is usually taken in large doses several times daily a few days prior to competition. By some indications, phosphate loading increases the oxygen-carrying capacity of the blood and makes more glucose available to the working muscles—two pluses if you're a competitive athlete.

But most of us aren't, so be forewarned: Phosphate loading isn't for regular exercisers or even moderately active people. It can cause vomiting, upset the body's electrolyte balance, and lead to other untoward reactions. Despite the research supporting its benefits, phosphate loading is risky, so stay away from it.

Bioflav-
onoids

Bioflavonoids are a group of natural pigments that produce the colors of many flowers, fruits, and vegetables. They range from pale yellow in citrus fruit to red and blue in berries and are usually concentrated in the skin, peel, and outer layers of fruits and vegetables. Tea, coffee, wine, and beer also contain significant amounts of bioflavonoids.

Claims for the use of bioflavonoids include prevention or treatment of high blood pressure, degenerative vascular disease, rheumatic fever, arthritis, cancer, and other diseases. None of these claims has been verified by research, although bioflavonoids have been used pharmaceutically for the treatment of blood clotting and hemorrhage.

On average, we ingest about 1,000 mg of bioflavonoids daily in our diets, and a typical supplement tablet contains a mere 20 to 30 mg. Supplement pills may contain the cancer-causing bioflavonoid quercetin and should be avoided. Get your bioflavonoids from food.

Fish Oil
Supplements

Scientists have recently discovered that certain types of oils from fish and shellfish, called omega-3 fatty acids, have protective benefits against heart disease, strokes, and blood clotting. This discovery has prompted some nutritionists to recommend more fish, especially fatty fish like salmon, in the diet. That's a recommendation I support.

But I don't recommend using fish oil supplements. You can get the same protection by eating two to three fish or shellfish meals each week. An excess of these oils can be harmful and cause internal or external bleeding. Being a fat, they're high in calories, and that can promote weight gain. Unregulated, fish oil supplements are rarely pure and often contain concentrations of highly toxic elements.

MCT Oil

Another oil you may have heard about is medium-chain triglyceride oil (MCT oil), usually processed from coconut oil. This special dietary fat was first formulated in the 1950s by the pharmaceutical industry for patients who had trouble digesting regular fats. Still used in medical settings, MCT oil is also a popular fitness supplement, marketed as a fat burner, muscle builder, and energy source.

Because of its unique chemical makeup, fatty acids in MCT oil are digested, transported, and metabolized much more quickly than fatty acids from regular oils or fats. MCTs are used immediately for energy, sparing blood glucose. Interestingly, MCT oil is burned in the body like a carbohydrate, so it's not stored as easily as fat calories are.

But can it help you burn body fat, as some have claimed? Most of the research showing that it may has been done on rats. This has led some to suggest that MCT oil may have an important role in the prevention and control of obesity in humans. That's stretching the research a bit, so I wouldn't place too much stock in MCT oil as a fat burner just yet.

Another claim attached to MCT oil is that it helps you put on muscle. But no controlled studies have been done to prove this. Using some MCT oil to sneak in extra calories for harder workouts makes some sense, though. But don't go over-board. MCT oil contains roughly 114 calories a tablespoon. Too many calories from MCT oil, like any food, will turn into fat on your body. Go easy at first by taking a half a tablespoon to a tablespoon a day. Its fast absorption can cause cramping and diarrhea if you eat too much.

If you decide to experiment with MCT oil, check with your doctor first. Use the supplement only while following a high-carbohydrate diet. If carbs are in short supply, MCT oil can cause ketosis, a condition in which by-products of fat metabolism called ketones build up in the body because carbs aren't available to assist in the final stages of fat breakdown.

Lecithin and Choline

Lecithin is a fat found in nervous tissue, primarily the myelin sheath (the protective covering for the nerves); in egg yolk, soybeans, and corn; and as an essential constituent of animal and vegetable cells. It helps emulsify cholesterol in the body. As a supplement, lecithin comes in capsules, granules, and liquid form.

Lecithin is the richest source of choline, a nutrient that prevents fats from building up in the liver and aids the body in metabolizing cholesterol. Choline also shuttles fats into cells to be used for energy. Your body can easily manufacture enough choline for good health as long as you eat a balanced, nutrient-rich diet. Choline is found in eggs, fish, soybeans, liver, brewer's yeast, and wheat germ. There's no established daily requirement for choline because it's so readily available from food. Even if you ate a choline-deficient diet, your body can still manufacture it from the amino acid methionine.

Choline's role as a cholesterol and fat dissolver in the body has given it a reputation as a *lipotropic,* or fat-burning, agent. Because lecithin is so full of choline, it too has been dubbed a fat burner. For years, both nutrients have found their way into supplement formulations marketed as fat burners.

Taking lecithin and choline as supplements doesn't burn fat, however, since the nutrients are metabolized as food would be. To date there's no single magic pill or potion that will burn fat, regardless of how creatively the product is hyped. Nor does any research exist to support the fat-burning claims of lecithin and choline used in supplemental form.

Although choline has long been thought of as a fat burner, it has recently been touted as a new wonder nutrient for athletes and exercisers. The reason has to do with the fact that choline is a constituent of acetylcholine in the body. Acetylcholine is a *neurotransmitter.* Neurotransmitters are chemicals that send messages from nerves to nerves and nerves to muscles. When muscles reach a fatigue point during exercise, this transmission system gets blocked. No messages are sent, and muscular work slows down or ceases temporarily.

Researchers at MIT studied runners before and after the Boston Marathon and found a 40 percent drop in their plasma choline concentrations. They don't know why this happened; however, they speculated that choline is used up during exercise to produce the neurotransmitter acetylcholine. Once choline is depleted, there's a corresponding drop in acetylcholine production. When production falls off, the ability to do muscular work falls off, too. Or so the theory goes. Only a handful of studies have been done on choline and exercise. To date there's just not enough information to suggest that choline supplementation enhances performance.

Bee Pollen and Royal Jelly

Bee pollen became the rage in the 1980s when then-President Reagan attributed his youthful vigor to daily doses of the supplement. You may be surprised to learn that the product sold as bee pollen is actually a loose powder of bee saliva, plant nectar, and pollen compressed into tablets of 400 to 500 mg or poured into capsules. It also comes in pellets to be sprinkled on foods. Often bee pollen is formulated with other supplements.

Bee pollen is rich in amino acids, with a protein content that averages 20 percent but ranges from 10 to 36 percent. Ten to 15 percent is simple sugars. There are traces of fats and minerals in bee pollen.

So many curative powers have been attached to it that you'd think bee pollen was a cure-all. But like most controversial and unproven supplements, there's no scientific proof behind any of the claims.

Bee pollen has also been marketed as an athletic supplement for improving physical performance. Some European studies find benefits, but American studies do not. Much of the disagreement rests on the design of the experiments. Most studies use pure sources of pollen extract from a single manufacturer, and these are not available to the average consumer.

Can bee pollen hurt you? Possibly. It does contain pollen, so you could have an allergic reaction if you're prone to allergies. Because of its high amino acid content, people with signs of gout or kidney disease should stay away from bee pollen.

Royal jelly is a milky white substance produced by worker bees. It's fed to the bee destined to become the queen bee. In fact, the feeding of royal jelly is what turns an ordinary bee into a queen bee—an insect that's larger, more fertile, and longer-lived. Advocates of royal jelly say it does the same for us—a far-fetched claim, to say the least. We aren't bees, so any preventive, therapeutic, or rejuvenating benefits of royal jelly can't be applied to humans.

Sold in capsules, royal jelly is a rich source of pantothenic acid, a B-complex vitamin involved in releasing energy from foods and in protecting against cellular damage. You can also get pantothenic acid from whole grain cereals. I see no reason to supplement with royal jelly when you can get the same nutritive value from everyday foods.

Some supplement manufacturers formulate their products with propolis, a resin collected by bees from the buds of trees, mixed with their wax, and used to line beehives. In 1994 one manufacturer had to recall all of its nutritional supplements containing propolis because it was thought to be contaminated with lead, which is toxic.

Inosine and Adenine

Inosine and adenine are chemical compounds found in RNA and DNA, both nucleic acids that carry genetic information. As supplements, they're promoted as energy boosters. This is because they naturally occur in ATP (adenosine triphosphate), the cellular fuel source produced by carbohydrates, fats, and amino acids for powering muscular activity.

Research has looked into whether inosine and adenine truly enhance energy. The studies, however, have been conducted on ill patients taking the compounds intravenously. Taken by mouth, inosine and adenine are broken down into products that may damage the intestinal lining and increase the risk of gout, a type of arthritis caused by too much uric acid in the blood. I strongly discourage the use of these products as supplements.

Coenzyme Q_{10} (Ubiquinone)

At the molecular level, this nutrient plays a central role in a series of chemical reactions that produce energy. It may also act as an antioxidant capable of disarming free radicals.

Supplementing with coenzyme Q_{10} to improve energy and performance has been hotly debated, but I find no conclusive proof of its benefit. In one study, trained triathletes took 100 mg of coenzyme Q_{10}, 500 mg of vitamin C, 100 mg of inosine, and 200 IU of vitamin E for four weeks. No change in their endurance capacity was found. A few studies have shown that coenzyme Q_{10} may enhance aerobic performance in people who don't exercise. All in all, there just isn't enough data to recommend supplementation with coenzyme Q_{10}.

Wheat Germ, Wheat Germ Oil, and Octacosanol

At the heart of a kernel of wheat grain is the germ, or the sprouting portion, of the kernel. It's an excellent source of vitamin E, protein, B-complex vitamins, and various minerals, including calcium, magnesium, phosphorus, copper, and manganese. Wheat germ is usually removed from the grain during milling because its fat content can turn the flour rancid. Wheat germ oil is extracted from wheat germ and sold as a nutritional supplement. It's also high in vitamin E.

From wheat germ oil comes the supplement octacosanol, an alcohol derivative of the oil. Athletes have long used octacosanol in the belief that it will improve energy, strength, and reaction time. Some studies have found a link between wheat germ oil or octacosanol supplementation and improvement in conditioned reflexes. But so far no research has turned up any proof that these supplements directly improve endurance or physical performance.

Using wheat germ, wheat germ oil, or octacosanol has no known adverse reactions or side effects. In fact, wheat germ is an excellent, nutrient-packed food to include in the diet, although it's rather high in calories (360 calories in a 3½-oz. serving).

Brewer's Yeast

Brewer's yeast, or nutritional yeast, is a rich source of B vitamins, especially vitamin B_{12}, and can be used as a vitamin B-complex supplement. It's also high in amino acids, minerals, and other vitamins. Proponents of brewer's yeast claim it's a panacea for heart trouble, aging, and other ailments, but no scientific evidence exists to support such claims.

Rely on Food

Stay on guard the next time you read about the latest magic bullet for athletes and exercisers. Put food first in your nutrition program. Relying on supplements over food is like outfitting your car with air bags, then driving too fast on the wrong side of the road. Even if you packed three hundred nutrients into a single pill, you would never get the same benefits as you would from food.

CHAPTER 13

Herbal Supplements

Adaptogens

Herbal products are an old breed of supplements being marketed in a new way to exercisers, bodybuilders, and athletes as "adaptogens." Coined by a Soviet scientist in 1947, the word *adaptogen* refers to a class of agents that build resistance to physical stress. But in today's new fitness jargon, this definition has been stretched far beyond its original meaning. Now adaptogen is used to describe any herb that supposedly enhances performance, extends endurance, and stimulates the body's recovery power following exercise. Take the bait of these claims, and you're sure to be disappointed, for there's no evidence to support them.

What Is an Herb?

An herb is a plant or a part of a plant valued for its medicinal qualities, its aroma, or its taste. Herbs and herbal remedies have been around for centuries. Even Neanderthal humans used plants for healing purposes. About 30 percent of all modern drugs are derived from herbs. One of the best known is aspirin. In the early 1800s, its active ingredient, salicin, was isolated from white willow bark, an anti-inflammatory plant used for thousands of years. Salicin was later synthesized into a simpler form called salicylic acid. But both produced intolerable side effects, so scientists began searching for a less noxious version. After years of work, a German scientist was finally able to modify salicylic acid into what we now know as aspirin.

Medical history is filled with herb-turned-remedy stories. Digitalis, an important drug used to treat congestive heart failure, was discovered two hundred years ago from an ingredient in foxglove, a common garden flower grown in England. Quinidine, an important cardiac drug, and its relative quinine, long used to treat malaria, both come from the bark of the Peruvian cinchona tree. Another bark-derived drug, taxol, now shows promise as a powerful cancer-fighting drug. You may also be familiar with psyllium, the seed of the fleawort plant that is the active ingredient in many natural laxative products and cereals. Even today pharmaceutical companies are scouring rain forests and other primitive locales to find native remedies and botanicals that may hold the cures for modern diseases.

Natural, but Not Always Safe

It's a common but dangerous notion to think that because herbs are natural, they are safe. Makers of herbal supplements in the United States don't have to submit their products to the Federal Drug Administration (FDA), so there's no regulation of product quality or safety. Without the enforcement of standards, you have a meager chance that the contents and potency described on labels are accurate.

At present, herbs in the United States are classified as food supplements. Labeling them as medicines would require stringent testing to prove their safety and effectiveness. This costs millions of dollars per herb, an investment few manufacturers are willing to make, especially since herbs can't be patented.

Herbs for Weight Loss

For the fitness conscious, a potentially dangerous lure of herbs lies in those supplements promising weight loss. A case in point: As reported in *The Lancet*, two women under the age of fifty had been following a slimming regimen prescribed by a weight loss clinic in Brussels, Belgium, when they were diagnosed with a type of "fibrosing interstitial nephritis." This is a kidney disease that can lead to kidney failure. Sadly, both women succumbed to it.

Medical investigators surveyed all the kidney dialysis units in Brussels and found seven more women with this disease, all of whom had attended the same clinic and followed the same weight loss program. Further investigation revealed that all nine women developed kidney problems after the clinic changed its weight loss formula to include two Chinese herbs: *Stephania tetrandra* and *Magnolia officinalis.*

Potential Dangers in Herbal Products

Potential dangers are lurking in herbal preparations. Unlike medicines, herbal dosages are not carefully prescribed, nor are herbs regulated. Consuming herbs in large amounts makes them doubly dangerous. If you take a medicine prescribed by a doctor and you have a bad reaction, you can pinpoint the cause and return to your doctor for help. In the case of a bad reaction to an herb, you may not figure it out so easily or know how to cure it.

I don't want to bash all herbal products. Many, like the herbal teas available in grocery and health food stores, are excellent caffeine-free beverages if you're trying to cut down on coffee and tea. There are medicinal herbs that can be appropriately prescribed for specific medical conditions. Capsaicin, for instance, made from hot peppers, is used in muscle rubs to create a very effective topical analgesic for sore muscles and joints. But beyond those uses, herbal products and supplements have little value to exercisers and athletes. In many cases, they may be harmful.

What follows is a rundown of fourteen well-known herbs, either sold alone or found in fitness supplements as part of the formulation. Keep in mind that most of these herbs are medically unproven.

Buchu

These dry leaves are usually sold as tea. Buchu is a mild diuretic and has some antiseptic (germ-fighting) properties. It is generally safe.

Burdock

This relative of the dandelion was used by the ancient Greeks as a healing remedy and throughout the Middle Ages as an important medicine. Researchers have isolated certain constituents of burdock that may fight bacteria and fungus.

A dried root usually sold as a tea, burdock is often called a blood purifier, a diuretic, a treatment for skin diseases like acne and psoriasis, and a diaphoretic (sweat producer). None of these claims has been verified scientifically, and no solid evidence exists that burdock has any useful therapeutic activity. The herb seems safe, although there have been reports of poisonings caused by burdock tea contaminated with the harmful herb belladonna.

Canaigre

Any herbal product marketed as wild red American ginseng or wild red desert ginseng is actually an herb called canaigre. But in no way is it related to ginseng, either botanically or chemically. The herb is deceptively promoted as a less expensive American alternative to bona fide ginseng.

Native to the southwestern United States and Mexico, canaigre has been recommended by herbal enthusiasts for a variety of problems, ranging from lack of energy to leprosy. The trouble is, canaigre is potentially cancer-causing due to its high content of tannin. I can think of no rational reason to use canaigre therapeutically. There's another side to the herb, though: It's useful for tanning leather and dyeing wool.

Damiana

Damiana comes from the leaves of a Mexican shrub. Around the turn of the century, it was touted as a powerful aphrodisiac. But any such effects were actually caused by the presence of other drugs in the preparation. Closer scientific scrutiny of damiana revealed that it has no aphrodisiac properties or any beneficial physiological action whatsoever.

Ephedra (Ma Huang)

Ephedra, a short-acting stimulant also known as ma huang, is the world's oldest known cultivated plant. For more than five thousand years, it has been grown in China for the treatment of respiratory diseases. Two familiar medicinal compounds are synthesized from it: ephedrine, used to treat bronchial asthma, and pseudoephedrine, found in nasal decongestants such as Sudafed.

Both compounds stimulate the central nervous system. When taken in excessive doses, they can cause sleeplessness, anxiety, and nervousness. Ephedrine is especially potent. It can make the heart race and blood pressure soar. Because of these adverse effects, people with heart conditions, high blood pressure, or diabetes should stay away from ephedrine.

A few years ago, the *Western Journal of Medicine* documented a case in which a woman seeking relief for an upper respiratory infection turned to a Chinese herbalist for help. She was given two Chinese herbal concoctions. A day later she came down with a skin condition called erythroderma. This produces an intense burning sensation on the skin, a widespread rash, and exfoliation or peeling of the skin. Later tests revealed that both herbal preparations contained ephedrine.

Chemically, ephedrine resembles our body's own stimulant, adrenaline, which, among other functions, liberates fat from cells to be used as energy. For this reason, the herb ephedra is found in many herbal remedies marketed for weight loss. Studies in Denmark showed that a drug made of ephedrine and caffeine helped to promote weight loss; however, the combination produced central nervous system side effects such as agitation.

When abused, ephedra and its active compound ephedrine can be lethal. In 1993 neurologists from the University of New Mexico reported that ephedrine had caused strokes in three people who had exceeded the recommended dosages.

Ephedrine made the headlines during the World Cup soccer competition in 1994 when Argentina soccer star Diego Maradona apparently tested positive for the drug during random testing that summer. Ephedrine is one of many drugs banned in international competition. Allegedly, Maradona's urine sample contained four other banned drugs besides ephedrine: norephedrine, pseudoephedrine, norpseudoephedrine, and methephedrine. Like ephedrine, all are stimulants. Since no medication contains all five substances, medical officials concluded that Maradona had taken a drug cocktail.

According to the Drug Enforcement Administration (DEA), ephedrine is being used to make a powerful—and illegal—new street drug known as methocathinone, or "cat." It produces a high that lasts seven to fourteen hours. Users get paranoid, hyperactive, and lose their appetite. Dangerous amounts of weight can be lost.

When taken in small, recommended doses as part of a cold remedy, ephedrine seems safe. But other dangers lurk if you take too much—like combining a decongestant with a weight loss preparation. I advise that you avoid any herbal preparation containing ephedra, since you don't know how much ephedrine is in the formula, or how your body will react to the drug.

Fo-ti

Ancient Chinese herbalists swear that this member of the buckwheat family is one of the best longevity promoters ever grown. As they see it, fo-ti exhibits different properties depending on the size and age of its root. A fist-size fifty-year-old plant, for example, keeps your hair from turning gray. A hundred-year-old root the size of a bowl preserves your cheerfulness. At 150 years old and as large as a sink, fo-ti makes your teeth fall out so that new ones can grow in. And a two-hundred-year-old plant restores youth and vitality. Or so the folktales go.

Fo-ti also has a reputation as a good cardiovascular herb. Supposedly it lowers cholesterol, protects blood vessels, and increases blood flow to the heart. But these claims can't be backed up scientifically. Fo-ti does act as a laxative, however. It's probably a safe herb in that regard.

Garlic and Alliums

Wear garlic around your neck, and you're sure to ward off vampires—or so the ghost stories go. Today garlic claims to ward off heart disease and cancer.

Garlic and its relatives—onions, leeks, scallions, and shallots (the allium family)—have been getting a lot of attention lately, thanks to some new studies hinting at the healing power in these foods. Much of the focus is on garlic's cholesterol-lowering potential.

The possible connection between garlic and cholesterol came to light a number of years ago when researchers studied the vegetarian diets of three groups of people in India. Of the three groups, the people who ate the most garlic and onions—about 1¾ oz. of garlic and ⅓ lb. of onions a week—had the lowest cholesterol. Those who ate no garlic or onions had the highest.

More recently, a study published in the *Annals of Internal Medicine* found that eating the equivalent of a half to a whole clove of garlic each day for eight to forty-two days cut total cholesterol levels by about 9 percent. Subjects took the pungent herb in the form of garlic tablets, powder, or a liquid extract.

The American Heart Association (AHA) called the reduction "modest" when compared with the effect of cholesterol-reducing drugs. As the AHA further pointed out, eating healthy servings of soluble fiber such as oat bran produces the same reduction as garlic does.

The spotlight is also on the cancer-fighting properties of garlic and onions. In China, for example, there's less stomach cancer in people who eat a lot of garlic. Here's the probable reason: Garlic and onions contain phytochemicals called *allylic sulfides*. These activate enzymes inside cells that disarm cancer-causing chemicals. The medical possibilities have aroused notice at the National Cancer Institute, where garlic studies are already in progress.

If there's a message in all of this, it's that garlic and onions are healthy foods to include or increase in your diet. Eating them raw is best, since this preserves the protective substances inside. Garlic, onions, and other alliums, however, shouldn't be looked upon as heal-alls or cures for cancer, heart disease, and other life-threatening conditions.

Ginseng

Ginseng was discovered in New England in the early eighteenth century. By the late 1700s, this American variety (*Panax quinquefolius*) was exported to China, eventually becoming a cash crop by the mid-nineteenth century.

There are several other types of ginseng. One is the native Asian variety, known as Panax ginseng. A lesser-known yet related type is Japanese ginseng, or Panax japonicus. You may have also heard of "Siberian ginseng," or eleuthero ginseng. Its active components are different from the others, and it is not a member of the Panax classification.

The American and Asian varieties are the two major types of ginseng, and both have similar chemical makeups. Nearly 2,900 scientific studies have been conducted on ginseng, mainly the Asian variety. In China today many preparations of ginseng are officially approved for medicinal use.

Ginseng has a reputation as an aphrodisiac, an adaptogen, an anabolic (tissue builder), and an antioxidant. There's no proof that ginseng enhances sexual performance or potency. But some evidence suggests that it may positively influence stress. Animal studies show some tissue-building reaction to ginseng taken orally; however, researchers haven't been able to replicate those results in humans.

The American and Asian plants contain active compounds called ginsenosides. Some research shows that ginsenosides may halt the buildup of plaque in the arteries and reduce cancer risk by preventing cell damage caused by oxidation.

Of interest to exercisers and athletes is ginseng's possible effect on performance. Italian researchers recently investigated the stamina-producing powers of ginseng. They studied fifty male sports teachers, all healthy, ages twenty-one to forty-seven. Every six weeks the participants took two capsules containing ginseng extract, vitamins, and minerals. Some participants were given placebos. After taking either the ginseng preparation or the placebo, they exercised on a treadmill at increasing workloads. The ginseng group performed much better than the placebo subjects. This finding led the researchers to conclude that the ginseng preparation boosted work capacity by improving the subjects' supply of oxygen to the muscles.

You find ginseng in teas and as powders, capsules, extracts, tablets, and ginseng-flavored soft drinks, yet many of these products are of variable quality and content. Authentic, high-grade ginseng is expensive, often costing as much as $20 an ounce. That being so, less ethical manufacturers have been known to dilute their products or use fillers in them. It's difficult to know what you're getting.

In my opinion, taking ginseng is a questionable practice. Large doses and long-term use have known side effects: high blood pressure, nervousness, insomnia, low blood pressure, sedation, painful breasts, breast nodules, and vaginal bleeding. Proof of ginseng's reported benefits is still sketchy. Until more studies are done in the United States, I'd leave this herb on the shelves.

Gotu Kola

Legend has it that if you eat a leaf of gotu kola every day, you'll live to be one thousand! Gotu kola is a common weed, usually found growing in drainage ditches in Asia and orchards in Hawaii. A member of the parsley family, it's reputed to be an aphrodisiac, a memory restorative, and a wound healer. As you might guess, no evidence supports these claims. No reputable medical expert knows if gotu kola is even safe to use.

Guarana

If you see pills in the health food store promising pep and vitality, they probably contain guarana, a dry paste made from crushed plant seeds. Marketed as an energy-giving aid, guarana is a stimulant—but only because it contains a lot of caffeine. Popping a few guarana pills gives you the same kick as a 50-cent cup of coffee.

Maté

Another caffeine-containing herb is maté, dried leaves that come as a tea. It too is advertised as a natural pep producer. But any stimulating effects are only the result of the herb's 2 percent caffeine content.

Pau d'Arco

The name refers to the bark of various species of trees. As an herbal agent, pau d'arco is found as a tea or in cosmetic preparations. It's often billed as a cancer cure. Indeed, the bark contains a tiny amount of lapachol, an agent shown in research to have anticancer properties. But when given in therapeutic doses, lapachol produces unbearable side effects.

Other disease-fighting benefits have been attributed to pau d'arco, but all are unproven. Pau d'arco is potentially toxic and not to be fooled with.

Sassafras

Usually found as a tea, this well-known herb sounds like a cure-all. It has been promoted as a stimulant, a muscle relaxant, a sweat producer, a blood purifier, and a treatment for rheumatism, skin diseases, and typhus. None of these benefits has been supported or even documented by medical science.

Even if there were some therapeutic effect, it could come with a deadly price. Sassafras contains safrole, an oil once used in root beer. This oil is cancer-causing, as are other agents in sassafras. So it's little wonder that sassafras and safrole were banned by the FDA in the early 1960s for use as flavors or food additives. Because of its harmful properties, I wouldn't recommend that sassafras tea be consumed at all, not even in small amounts or weak concentrations.

Saw Palmetto

Saw palmetto, an herb sold as the ripe or dried berries of the fan palm, has an interesting background. In Germany it's one of several plants approved to help men with benign prostatic hypertrophy (BPH), an enlargement of the prostate gland. Purportedly, saw palmetto helps increase urinary flow, cuts the frequency of urination, and makes it easier to pass urine. Several herbal medicines containing saw palmetto are marketed in Europe.

In 1990, the FDA banned all over-the-counter preparations used to treat BPH, including saw palmetto. Now you find it only for use as a tea. Even so, the herb has some wild claims attached to it. It's marketed to build bust size, heighten the sex drive, increase sperm production, reverse testis and breast shrinkage, and relieve the soreness of inflamed membranes in the urinary tract.

When saw palmetto was injected into young female mice, their estrogen activity—the hormone responsible for development of breasts and other secondary sex characteristics—speeded up. But taking saw palmetto by mouth is another matter. Its active ingredients dissolve in water. What's more, the body doesn't absorb saw palmetto well. So there's no real therapeutic benefit.

Some Cautions

As you can probably tell, using herbal supplements has no real place in a nutrition program for athletes and exercisers. My advice: If you take herbal supplements, do so sparingly and with caution. Anyone who is pregnant should not use herbs. Do not give herbs to children. If you take medication, consult a physician, pharmacist, or nutritionist before using any herbal supplement.

For the most credible information about herbs as medicines, read *Herbs of Choice* by Varro E. Tyler, Ph.D., Sc.D. (Pharmaceutical Products Press, 1994).

CHAPTER 14

Caffeine

Caffeine as a Drug

You know caffeine best as the ingredient in your coffee and tea that gets you going in the morning, but did you also know it's used as a supplement to enhance endurance? That's because caffeine temporarily reduces fatigue, increases alertness, and boosts muscle capacity. But what most people who use it forget is that caffeine is a drug—in fact, the most widely used drug in the world. That being the case, is it a good idea to use caffeine if your goal is to be healthy, fit, and active? Does using caffeine conflict with a fitness-oriented lifestyle? Here's a look at how caffeine affects performance and health.

Physical Reactions to Caffeine

Caffeine is a common ingredient in coffee and tea, as well as in other foods, soft drinks, and medications. (See tables 14-1 and 14-2 for a complete listing.) Even decaffeinated coffee has traces of caffeine. If you drink a lot of decaf, the amount of caffeine you take in can really pile up. Caffeine is also found in nonprescription diet medications, and one reason for including it is that the drug accelerates the metabolic rate by as much as 16 percent.

As a drug, caffeine is classified as a central nervous system stimulant. It makes your heart beat faster. It gives you that wide-awake feeling, too, sometimes bordering on the jitters, depending on how much you take. Blood levels of caffeine peak about thirty to sixty minutes after taking it.

How you react to its power is highly individual, depending on your body composition, age, usage patterns, and the amount you take. Young children, for example, are highly sensitive to the stimulating effects of caffeine. Just one can of caffeinated cola (45 mg) in a child can be as stimulating as a whole mug of coffee (275 mg) in an adult.

Table 14-1

CAFFEINE CONTENT OF BEVERAGES AND FOODS

Beverages and Foods	Range (mg)
Coffee (5-oz. cup)	
Brewed, drip method	110–150
Brewed, percolator	64–124
Instant	40–108
Decaffeinated, brewed or instant	2–5
Tea (5-oz. cup)	
Brewed, 1 minute	9–33
Brewed, 3 minutes	20–46
Brewed, 5 minutes	20–50
Instant tea	12–28
Iced tea (12-oz. glass)	22–36
Cocoa (5-oz. cup)	
Made from mix	6
Milk chocolate (1 oz.)	6
Baking chocolate	35
Chocolate milk beverage (8 oz.)	2–7
Soft drinks (12-oz. can)	
Mountain Dew	54
Mello Yellow	52
Tab	46
Coca Cola, Diet Coke	46
Shasta Cola	44
Dr. Pepper, Mr. Pibb	40
Sugar-free Dr. Pepper	40
Pepsi Cola	38
Diet Pepsi	36
Pepsi Light	36

*Source:*Adapted from A. R. Wilcox, "Caffeine and Endurance Performance," *Gatorade Sports Science Exchange* 3, no. 26 (1990): 3.

Table 14-2

CAFFEINE CONTENT OF OVER-THE- COUNTER DRUGS

*Drugs	Caffeine (mg)
Cold remedies (standard dose)	
Dristan	0
Coryban-D	30
Triaminicin	30
Diuretics (standard dose)	
Aqua-ban	100
Pre-Mens Forte	100
Pain relievers (standard dose)	
Aspirin, plain (any brand)	0
Anacin	32
Excedrin	65
Midol	32
Vanquish	33
Stimulants	
No Doz	100
Vivarin	200
Weight control aids (daily dose)	
Dexatrim	200
Prolamine	140
Prescription pain relievers	
Cafergot	100
Darvon compound	32
Fiorinal	40
Migralam	100

*Source:*Adapted from: A. R. Wilcox, "Caffeine and Endurance Performance," *Gatorade Sports Science Exchange* 3, no. 26 (1990): 3.

*Because products change, contact the manufacturer for updates.

After drinking a cup of coffee, you feel alert. You can think more clearly, and you're not as tired. Caffeine stays in the body for a while, meaning that even small amounts can build up over time. Four to six hours after you drink your morning cup, only half the amount of the caffeine in it is metabolized by your body. This is called the half-life of the drug. If you're taking oral contraceptives, the half-life increases to ten hours; if you're a smoker, it decreases by an hour.

Caffeine's half-life can become counterproductive. By drinking small amounts through the day, you eventually reach a point at which your body has more than it can handle. You feel less wide awake, edgy, even anxious. Some people even complain of stomach upset from the stimulating action of caffeine on the secretion of stomach acids. Some other unwanted side effects include irritability, headaches, and diarrhea.

Other more serious complications have been associated with caffeine. It's thought to cause changes in the breasts of women with fibrocystic breast disease, in which there are benign lumps in the breast. Pregnant women who drink more than 300 mg of caffeine a day put themselves at risk for aborting spontaneously or retarding their baby's growth. A nursing mother who consumes caffeine passes it through her breast milk to her baby, making the infant restless and agitated. Caffeine also inhibits the absorption of the B-complex vitamin thiamin, important for carbohydrate metabolism, and several minerals, including calcium and iron.

If you're a woman who drinks a mugful of coffee a day and doesn't take in enough calcium (i.e., you consume 600 mg a day or below), you're putting yourself in harm's way of getting osteoporosis. New research shows that coffee-drinking women with low-calcium diets have higher losses of calcium in their urine and weaker bones. These losses are greater in older women because younger women are better able to absorb calcium.

A Diuretic

If you're a coffee or tea drinker, you know that caffeine is a diuretic, meaning that it increases fluid losses from the body. In fact, caffeine can increase urination by as much as 30 percent for up to three hours after drinking it. This is a significant loss of water. If you think you're taking in enough fluids with several cups of coffee, think again. You're flushing too much water from your body and risking dehydration. Rather than rely on coffee or tea, get your fluids by drinking eight to ten glasses of water daily.

Performance Effects

Caffeine has long been used by athletes. Power athletes were among the first to exploit it, mainly to enhance short-term, intense exercise. But early studies of caffeine's effect on short-term, high-intensity exercise were not conclusive, because of differences in doses, the type of exercise tested and its intensity, the diets of subjects and their caffeine use, and other factors.

As for endurance competition, some researchers theorized that supplementing with caffeine might prolong exercise before exhaustion set in. The possible reason: exercise and caffeine mobilize fat for energy, sparing muscle glycogen (stored carbohydrate) to be used later. Also, caffeine may provide a psychological boost by making the work seem easier. Most of these early studies on caffeine and endurance were inconclusive as well.

In the last few years, several well-designed studies have helped clear up some of the confusion over caffeine. At the University of Guelph in Ontario, Dr. Larry Spriet and his colleagues looked into the effect of caffeine on power sports. In one study, fourteen exercisers did three bouts of exercise as hard as they could. Each bout was separated by six minutes of rest. The first two exercise bouts lasted two minutes each, and bout three was performed to exhaustion. The exercisers were tested twice, once with caffeine and once with a placebo. In bout three, they were able to exercise longer using caffeine (4.93 minutes with caffeine compared with 4.12 minutes with the placebo). Caffeine clearly boosted performance in short-term, intense exercise.

But how? The mechanism isn't exactly clear, but the researchers were able to rule out one possibility. By taking blood samples and muscle biopsies, they found that caffeine did not spare muscle glycogen, as was previously thought.

If you want the kick caffeine gives you for exercise, how much should you drink? In another study at the University of Guelph, eight subjects took a placebo, 3, 6, or 9 mg of caffeine per kilogram of body weight. An hour later, they ran at a moderately high intensity until exhaustion. The subjects who ingested 3 and 6 mg were able to run longer, compared with those who took the placebo. When 9 mg were taken, the subjects performed worse than they did while on the placebo. However, supplementing with 9 mg of caffeine per kilogram of body weight produced the greatest rise in metabolism as measured by blood samples.

To be sure of the results, the researchers repeated their tests. They concluded that 3 to 6 mg per kilogram of body weight does give you more staying power. That amount translates into about two to three cups of drip coffee for a 150-lb. person.

You'd think that habitual coffee drinkers and noncoffee drinkers would react differently to caffeine during exercise. Logically, it would seem that nonusers would be more sensitive and thus have a greater response to caffeine than regular users. However, this is not the case. Dr. Spriet's group studied people who went through zero, two, and four days of caffeine withdrawal prior to receiving a caffeine supplement for an exercise trial. The results showed that the days of withdrawal had no impact on exercise performance, suggesting that regular caffeine users get just as much of a jolt during exercise from caffeine supplementation as nondrinkers do.

Most of these studies have used well-trained athletes. But what about regular exercisers? When a group of sedentary men (their average age was twenty-four) was given 5 mg of caffeine prior to walking on a treadmill at low and moderate intensities for an hour, they experienced no benefit from supplementation.

Athletes and Caffeine

Today caffeine's popularity is growing among endurance athletes hoping to gain a competitive advantage in long races and among strength athletes who want to push harder in workouts. But despite the newer research, I still don't see much evidence to recommend its use as an endurance-enhancing supplement. In fact, using caffeine in this manner has plenty of drawbacks.

The large dosages used by athletes—the equivalent of eight to ten cups of coffee—can produce the jitters, ultimately harming performance. Such dosages are also illegal for Olympic competition—and detectable by drug testing.

As noted previously, caffeine is a diuretic, causing fluid loss. This should be of special concern if you're an athlete. Fluid losses can rapidly bring on dehydration, and performance can suffer. Caffeine also relaxes the muscles of the large intestine, so you might want to forgo the coffee before a race to make sure you don't get diarrhea during it.

Weigh the Risks

You're the best judge of how much coffee is enough for you. Caffeine may aggravate certain health problems, such as ulcers, heart disease, high blood pressure, and anemia, to name just a few. Stick to your doctor's advice. As far as regular exercise goes, I don't see any real value in trying to get a caffeine "buzz" on before you work out. Rely instead on sound, commonsense nutritional practices for extending energy.

PART FIVE

FLUID NEEDS
OF EXERCISERS

CHAPTER 15

Water

A Critical Nutrient

Water is a life-giving nutrient making up about 60 percent of your body weight. You can live up to forty days without food, but you'll die within a week without water. Athletes and exercisers need even more water than the average person.

The fluids in your body form a heavily trafficked river through your arteries, veins, and capillaries that carries nutrients to your cells and waste products away and out of the body. Fluids fill virtually every space in your cells and between them. Water molecules not only fill space, they help form the structures of macromolecules like proteins and glycogen. The chemical reactions that keep you alive occur in water, and water is an active participant in those reactions.

Water performs many other essential functions. As the primary fluid in your body, water serves as a solvent for minerals, vitamins, amino acids, glucose, and many other nutrients. Without water, you can't even digest these essential nutrients, let alone absorb, transport, and utilize them. And when your temperature begins to rise, water is to your body what coolant is to the radiator of your car.

Water Losses

Your body produces energy so it can live, breathe, and move. But only 25 percent of that energy is actually used for mechanical work. The other 75 percent is released as heat. During exercise, the extra heat produced raises your core temperature. To get rid of that heat, you sweat. As sweat evaporates, your blood and body get cold. That's good. Without this cooling-off ability, you'd quickly succumb to dangerous heat stress, a result of an increasing body core temperature.

A 150-pound man carries about 45 qt. of fluid in his body; a 120-pound woman, about 36 qt. With a sedentary lifestyle, the man loses about 3 qt. of fluid a day and the women about 2.5 qt. through perspiration and excretion. In the desert, he can lose more than 10 qt. of fluid in one day; the woman, more than 8 qt.

Water and Muscular Performance

Muscular movement depends on the presence of water. Water is found in highest concentration in metabolically active tissues like muscle, and in lowest amounts in relatively inactive tissues such as fat, skin, and some parts of bone. Muscles are controlled by nerves. The electrical stimulation of nerves and contraction of muscles occur due to the exchange of electrolyte minerals dissolved in water (sodium, potassium, calcium, chloride, and magnesium) across the nerve and muscle cell membranes. If you're low on water or electrolytes, muscle strength and control are weakened.

The heart is a muscle, too, and its function depends on electrical stimulation. The electrical impulses in our brain and balance mechanisms are also extremely sensitive to the presence of adequate water. Adequate water and electrolytes directly affect the proper functioning of these critical organ systems.

Water also forms the makeup of synovial fluid, the lubricating fluid between your joints, and cerebrospinal fluid, the shock-absorbing fluid between vertebrae and around the brain. Both fluids are essential for healthy joint and spine maintenance. If your diet is water-deficient, even for a brief period, less fluid is available to protect these areas. Strength training places tremendous demands on joints and spines, and the presence of adequate protective fluid is essential for optimum performance and long-term health.

Water and Fat Burning

Drinking more water can actually help you stay lean, indirectly. Your kidneys depend on enough water to do their job of filtering waste products from the body. In a water shortage, the kidneys need backup, so they turn to the liver for help. One of the liver's many functions is mobilizing stored fat for energy. By taking on extra assignments from the kidneys, the liver can't do its fat-burning job as well. Fat loss is compromised as a result.

Dehydration: The Warning Signs

Generally, most people just don't drink enough water and are less than 100 percent hydrated. Add exercise and warm climate on top of that, and you spell dehydration in bold letters. Are you at risk? Table 15-1 lists some warning signs of dehydration and heat stress.

Table 15-1

WARNING SIGNS OF DEHYDRATION AND HEAT STRESS

Early Signs	Severe Signs
Fatigue	Difficulty swallowing
Loss of appetite	Stumbling
Flushed skin	Clumsiness
Heat intolerance	Shriveled skin
Light-headedness	Sunken eyes and dim vision
Dark urine with a strong odor	Painful urination
	Numb skin
	Muscle spasm
	Delirium

It's easy to monitor yourself for early signs of dehydration:

- Your urine should be light colored with little odor. If it's a golden color or deep color with a strong odor, you're dehydrated.
- Sore throat, dry cough, and a hoarse voice are all other signs of dehydration.
- A burning sensation in your stomach can signal dehydration.
- Check your weight before and after exercise. Any weight loss during exercise is fluid loss and should be replaced by fluids as soon after exercise as possible.
- Watch for muscle cramps. No one knows for sure what causes muscle cramps, but dehydration may be at the root of the problem. Muscles cramp more easily when the body is in a drought. Sweat loss and dehydration can disrupt the balance between the electrolytes potassium and sodium, also leading to cramps. The muscle won't return to normal until fluid is replaced and electrolyte balance is restored.

Water Loss during Exercise

Depending on your size and how much you sweat, you lose about a quart of water (4 cups) per hour of exercise. If it's hot and humid, up to 2 qt. (8 cups) an hour drain from your body. For every pint or 2 cups of fluid lost, you lose a pound of water weight. Scientists define dehydration as fluid losses greater than just 1 percent of body weight.

For every 2.2 lb. (1 kg) of water lost during prolonged exercise in the heat:

- Your heart rate elevates about eight beats per minute.
- Cardiac output declines by 1 liter a minute.
- Your core temperature rises 0.3 degrees Celsius.

If our 150-pound man loses 2 percent of his body water (6 cups or 3 lb.), his athletic performance will drop by 20 percent. If he loses 4 percent of his body water (12 cups or 6 lb.), his performance will drop by 30 percent, and he'll be at risk for heat exhaustion.

Proper Hydration during Exercise

If you're sedentary, you need to drink a minimum of eight to ten 8-oz. glasses (2 qt.) of fluid every day. Exercisers need this minimum but must also replace the fluids lost during exercise. Don't depend on feeling thirsty to get you to the water fountain, either. Thirst is not nearly as powerful as hunger. What's more, the thirst mechanism is even less powerful during exercise. You must get yourself on a scheduled plan to drink often throughout the day.

It's important to remember that dehydration is cumulative. If you fail to re-hydrate on one day, your body can't rehydrate itself. The next day, you'll become even more dehydrated and begin to suffer from the early signs of dehydration.

At home and at work, I keep a water bottle nearby and take sips every ten minutes. This keeps me well hydrated. For workouts, here's a schedule that will keep you well-hydrated:

✔ *Before exercise:* Drink 8 to 16 oz. (1 to 2 cups) of fluid two hours before exercise. Then, drink 4 to 8 oz. (.5 cup to 1 cup) of fluid immediately before exercise. In very hot or cold weather, you need even more water: 12 to 20 oz. (1.5 to 2.5 cups) of fluid ten to twenty minutes before exercise. Exercising during cold weather elevates your body temperature, and you still lose water through perspiration and respiration.

✔ *During exercise:* Drink 4 to 8 oz. every fifteen to twenty minutes during exercise (8 oz. [1 cup] in extreme temperatures). Although this might seem tough at first, once you schedule it into your regular training routine, you'll quickly adapt to the feeling of fluid in your stomach. In fact, the fuller your stomach, the faster it will empty. Dehydration slows the rate that your stomach will empty. Make regular water breaks part of your training now.

✔ *After exercise:* This is the time to replace any fluid you've lost. Drink 2 cups of fluid for every pound of lost body weight.

Because I always harped on the importance of drinking water during exercise to my mother, she's the only person in her aerobics class who takes a water bottle to class. At age seventy-three, my mother gets in more than five vigorous aerobics sessions a week, three of them step classes. One of the reasons she can perform at such a high level is proper hydration.

Even Swimmers Must Rehydrate

I frequently work with swimmers who think they don't need to drink much water during training. After all, they're surrounded by water—how could they possibly sweat? That's a dangerous misconception, though. Swimmers lose fluids just like other exercisers but just don't feel the dampness of the sweat in the same way.

I recently did a little experiment on myself to check my own fluid losses while swimming. After weighing myself, I swam indoors at a moderate pace for twenty minutes. Then I dried myself off and jumped on the scales again. I had lost one whole pound! In only twenty minutes, 2 cups of fluid had drained from my body.

Many of you may swim or do water exercise. How can you drink while you swim? Place an easily identifiable water bottle on the deck at the edge of the lap lane. Using a sports watch or a clock/timer at the pool, come up for air and a fluid break at scheduled intervals. Unless you sip while swimming, you'll tire out sooner. Remember, fatigue is one of the earliest signs of dehydration.

Which Water Is the Best to Drink?

The most convenient choice is tap water straight from your faucet. Tap water contains a variety of minerals. In most cities, it's chlorinated and fluoridated. The mineral content in tap water varies regionally, and the amount of chlorine and fluoride added to water is federally and locally regulated.

There's been a lot of controversy about tap water lately. Two environmental reports issued in 1995 reported that 53 million Americans have been exposed to sickening contaminants in their drinking water, including lead, pesticides, and chlorine by-products that exceed federal limits. Because of ongoing concerns like these, many people choose to drink bottled water rather than risk drinking tainted water.

There are more than six hundred brands of bottled water, and over fifty brands of imported bottled water. The U.S. Food and Drug Administration (FDA) regulates the classification, labeling, and content of bottled water, and several types of bottled waters are available, depending on their source and their method of treatment. In table 15-2, you'll find a primer of various types.

Regardless of the process or the origin of the water, distilled, purified, distilled natural, and purified natural waters all result in an identical product once

Table 15-2

A DRINKING WATER PRIMER

Drinking water	Bottled water that has been obtained from an approved source and has undergone special treatment to bring it within the accepted standards for drinking water established by the U.S. Environmental Protection Agency.
Natural water	Bottled spring, mineral, artesian well, or well water that comes from an underground formation and is not derived from a municipal system of public water supply. Natural water has not been modified by blending with water from another source, or by the addition or deletion of dissolved solids, except as it relates to disinfection and filtration.
Spring water	Water derived from an underground formation from which the water flows naturally to the surface of the earth. "Spring water" meets the requirements of "natural water."
Well water	Bottled water from a hole bored, drilled, or otherwise constructed in the ground which taps the water of an aquifer. "Well water" meets the requirements of "natural water." One of the potential problems with natural, spring, and well waters is that they may be contaminated with pesticide or chemical residues from local farm groundwater runoff. Local bottlers do not necessarily filter their waters for these residues, and the FDA does not always inspect these plants frequently enough to inhibit the potential for contamination. Minerals are never removed from these waters.
Distilled water	Water that is purified through vaporization and is then condensed. Only water that has been steam distilled can be labeled "distilled water."
Purified water	Water that has been purified by reverse osmosis, distillation, or deionization.
Distilled natural water	Water from a natural source that has been passed through the distillation process. Also applies to "spring" and "well" waters processed in this manner.
Purified natural water	Water from a natural source that has been purified according to government standards.

they're bottled. Virtually all the minerals and other substances have been re-moved, leaving behind pure water. If you drink these primarily, check with your physician or dentist about fluoride supplements. For anyone seeking strict control over mineral and chemical intakes, I recommend any of the purified waters. Just remember to drink plenty and often!

CHAPTER 16

Sports Drinks

Special Fluids for Exercisers

If you're like most people I work with, you want to get stronger, leaner, more toned, or muscular. And you want to get there fast. Unfortunately, there aren't any shortcuts. But you can make progress a lot faster—provided you've got the staying power to make it through a workout without wilting or the energy to step up to a higher level of intensity. Put simply, the harder you exercise, the stronger and fitter you'll get, as long as you're fueling yourself properly. Here's where sports drinks—fluid-electrolyte solutions, carbohydrate supplements, and meal replacers—can help.

Endurance athletes have used these supplements for years—to extend endurance, boost their training power, and add extra energy-giving calories to their diets. In my work with athletes and exercisers of all types, I've found that sports drinks have a place in almost every active person's life. They should be as much a part of your training gear as walking shoes, weights, exercise machines, or aerobic equipment.

Fluid-Electrolyte Solutions

Fluid-electrolyte solutions are a concoction of water, carbohydrate, and electrolytes. Dissolved, electrolytes make up a salty sea in and around cells. They act like electrical charges. This lets them react with other minerals to conduct nerve impulses, to make muscles contract or relax, and to regulate the fluid balance inside and outside cells. In hard workouts or athletic competitions lasting an hour or longer, electrolytes can be lost through sweat.

Sodium is one of the major electrolytes in sports drinks. It helps shuttle water across the wall of the small intestine for absorption into the bloodstream. Another key electrolyte is potassium, a partner with sodium at the cellular level. Together they control fluid distribution on either side of cell walls.

The electrolyte chloride is also added to help your body better absorb fluid. Some sports drinks contain magnesium, too. It does its work inside cells, turning carbs and protein into fuel.

Fluid-electrolyte solutions do two things: replace water and electrolytes lost through sweat and supply a small amount of carbohydrate to the working muscles. Most drinks are formulated with about 6 to 10 percent of carbohydrate. The carb is either glucose, a simple sugar; fructose, a fruit sugar; sucrose, ordinary table sugar (a blend of glucose and fructose); maltodextrin, a complex carbohydrate derived from corn; or a combination of these.

Choosing the Best Solution

Does the type of carb in the drink make a difference? You bet. Researchers at the Exercise Physiology Laboratory at the Quaker Oats Company looked into this. They found that glucose and sucrose both boost performance, even in people who exercise for only an hour. But fructose didn't measure up as well. In fact, it impaired performance. That may be because fructose doesn't get into your system as fast as either glucose or sucrose, and this slows down the rate of fluid absorption. Without enough fluid, muscle cells can't keep up the energy-producing reactions that drive activity. Also, fructose isn't converted to muscle glycogen fast enough for use by working muscles.

The Fructose Story

Ever had a stomachache, cramps, or diarrhea after eating fruit? If so, you might have "fructose intolerance"—a sensitivity to the fructose in fruit, fruit juices, sports drinks, or products containing high-fructose corn syrup. When breast-feeding my daughter, I got concerned because she was having frequent bouts of diarrhea. A little detective work exposed the culprit. The frozen yogurt I had been eating was laced with high-fructose corn syrup.

About 10 to 15 percent of the people I work with are sensitive to fructose. Most have a mild intolerance, with symptoms like stomach upset, diarrhea, and bloating. In rare cases in which someone lacks the enzyme needed to digest fructose, the symptoms will be more severe: vomiting, hypoglycemia (low blood sugar), jaundice, or enlarged liver.

If you have a reaction to fructose, stay away from it, especially before exercise. Stomach and intestinal cramps can set in right after you eat it.

Another fructose alert: Researchers at the USDA Human Nutrition Research Center in North Dakota have discovered that high levels of fructose in the diet can keep the body from properly using copper, an important trace mineral. Among other functions, copper is necessary for healthy bone formation and maintenance. In studies of postmenopausal women, eating too much fructose promoted bone loss, particularly when the subjects' diets were low in copper. If you are a big juice drinker, beware of added high-fructose corn syrup. You could be taking in more than you think. Always read ingredient labels.

When to Take a Fluid-Electrolyte Solution

The main fluid-electrolyte supplement I use with my clients is Gatorade, because it fits their needs and has been formulated based on well-conducted research. One 8-oz. serving contains: 50 calories, 14 g of carbohydrate, 0 g of protein, 0 g of fat, 25 mg of potassium, 24 mg of phosphorus, 97 mg of chloride, and 110 mg of sodium. Other good products are on the market as well. Check their labels to see whether the formulations are similar to what I use and recommend.

The best time to polish off one of these drinks is during your workout or during any period of exertion, especially if you're exercising or working in hot weather. That's when fluid loss is greater than any other time of the year. You lose more electrolytes, too, although the concentration of these minerals in sweat gets weaker the fitter you are. You also burn more glycogen working out in the heat—another reason to quench your body with a sports drink. (See table 16-1 for other times to use a sports drink.)

Liquid Carbohydrate Supplements

Are you training more days per week but fizzling out too early each workout? Doing more aerobics but dragging more than you're jogging? Want to pack on some lean mass but can't eat enough to stoke the muscle-building fires?

Liquid carbohydrate supplements to the rescue. These are formulated with water, some electrolytes, but more carbohydrate than you'll find in the fluid-electrolyte solutions. Look for them in sporting goods stores and specialty sports stores such as bicycle shops.

The best time to use a carbohydrate supplement is during your workout or right after it. During exercise, a carb supplement can keep your blood sugar (glucose) from dipping. That way, you stay energized for the duration of your workout.

By the time your workout is over, you're carb-needy. That's because your muscles are low on glycogen. It's best to start replenishing glycogen within thirty minutes after exercising, when blood flow to the muscles is high. Glucose can then be taken up swiftly by the body to start the glycogen-making process.

It's easy to see why a liquid carbohydrate supplement makes sense as a post-workout pick-me-up. As a low-bulk snack, it's absorbed more rapidly than carbs from food, so it gets into your system faster. The faster you start replenishing glycogen, the faster your muscles will recover. Using a carb supplement after workouts is a good way to make up the glycogen deficit.

Carbohydrate Supplements Can Benefit Any Exercise Program

The idea of using carb supplements to benefit any exercise program isn't so surprising, really. True, most of the studies on sports drinks and carb supplements have been done on endurance athletes. But think about it: If you're like a lot of exercisers, you're probably working out one or more hours a day, including some intense, heart-pumping aerobics. The way I see it, there's not a big difference between the training intensities of exercisers who cross-train with aerobics and strength training and those who do endurance sports.

Take the Cleveland Browns, for example. During the preseason, they trained all-out, up to six hours a day, including weight training and practice. This heavy schedule made it tough to get in enough calories every day. So the carb supplement was a convenient way to sneak in the calories. Plus, it provided a great energy source at the same time.

Something else: I had the players drink a mixture of half Gatorade and half GatorLode (Gatorade's carbohydrate supplement). This had two benefits. First, some carbohydrate supplements can be very sweet. The best way to cut the sweetness is to dilute the beverage, either with water or with a fluid-electrolyte solution. Second, diluting the supplement can spare you from possible cramps.

Don't overdo, however. If you drink too much of your carbohydrate supplement, diluted or undiluted, you could inadvertently take in too many calories. A good rule of thumb is to drink no more than 300 calories from a fluid-electrolyte solution or a carbohydrate supplement in one workout session. A 12-oz. serving of GatorLode contains 280 calories; an 8-oz. serving of Gatorade, 50 calories. Don't use these supplements in place of food, either. They don't provide all the nutrients you need.

Meal Replacers

Too busy to squeeze in all the calories you need in a day? Then try a meal replacer. These products have been developed to reproduce as closely as possible the nutrition you would normally get from food. They contain protein from sources that are well absorbed by the body; carbohydrate, usually from corn starch and sucrose; fat from corn oil (a healthy source of dietary fat); minerals and electrolytes; and vitamins. GatorPro, the meal replacer from Gatorade, doesn't contain the milk sugar lactose, making it excellent for people who have lactose intolerance—the inability to digest milk sugar. Look for other products that are formulated this way to find the one that you like best.

One of the biggest drawbacks of meal replacers, however, is that they tend to taste like a "vitamin milkshake" because of their concentration of vitamins and minerals. To disguise that flavor, drink your meal replacer cold, mixed in a blender with crushed ice, strawberries, or bananas.

Many of the people I work with share one bad habit: They skip breakfast—a big problem for people on the go. They dash out of the house in the morning without taking time to eat. Breakfast truly is the most important meal of the day. It stokes your metabolic fires after they've died down overnight so you can burn calories the rest of the day. If you're in the habit of skipping breakfast, reach for a meal replacer in the morning. Quick and easy to fix, it gives you a meal's worth of nutrients in a glass—and more energy-boosting carbohydrates than you'll find in a typical instant breakfast drink.

Make Your Own Meal Replacer

You can also make your own meal replacer by fortifying any instant breakfast product. Blend together a small banana, 1 tablespoon peanut butter, and 1 cup of

Table 16-1

A GUIDE FOR USING LIQUID SUPPLEMENTS

Timing	Fluid Replacer	Carbohydrate Supplement	Meal Replacer
Two or more hours before exercise or physical work*		8–16 oz.	8–16 oz.
Just before exercise or physical work	4–6 oz.		
During exercise or physical work	4–8 oz. every 15 to 20 minutes		
After exercise or physical work	8–16 oz.	12–24 oz. within 30 minutes	8 oz.
With meals		12 oz.	8 oz.
Between meals		12–24 oz.	8 oz.

Source: Adapted from The Scientific Basis of Training, Nutrition, and Athletic Performance. Brochure from the Gatorade Sports Science Institute.

*If solid food is unavailable or to add extra carbohydrates and calories to the diet.

nonfat milk with one serving of any flavor of Carnation Instant Breakfast powder. This is an economical way of getting in your morning nutrients and is the same recipe I use for my homemade firming formula. One serving supplies 438 calories, 17 g of protein, 70 g of carbohydrate, and 9 g of fat.

Remember, meal replacers should be used only as a *supplement* to your diet, not as a substitute for every meal. If you use them to replace food completely, you're headed for nutritional poverty. Occasional use, when you're going to miss a meal, is fine, and then you might want to drink two at a time, rather than one. Otherwise, use them primarily for increasing your caloric intake and feeding the muscles. GatorPro (Gatorade's meal replacer), for example, contains 360 calories in each 11-oz. serving. If you drink one of these each day for a week, you'll easily obtain the 2,500 extra calories you need for the energy to build a pound of lean muscle. Table 16-1 provides some guidelines for when to use liquid supplements.

Protein Powder

A popular protein supplement on the market is protein powder. These products are typically formulated with milk and egg protein or soy protein and contain small amounts of other ingredients such as carbohydrate (maltodextrin, glucose, sucrose, or fructose), vitamins, minerals, and electrolytes.

I feel strongly that protein powders are not needed in an active person's diet. You should get all the protein you need by following my nutrition recommendations and menus in appendix A. Consider supplementation with a protein powder only if you're not getting the recommended levels of protein suggested in chapter 5.

By far, the best and least expensive way to get supplemental protein is to use nonfat dry milk powder and add it to other foods such as cereal, soup, casseroles, and fruit juices. Four tablespoons of dry powder contains 10.9 g of high-quality protein, 15.6 g of carbohydrate, 0.2 g of fat, and 109 calories. Commercial protein powder or nonfat powdered milk can be used to replace the protein from one meal each day, and no more.

Protein powders formulated with soy protein can be used in vegetarian diets as well, if you can't get in enough protein with food. When supplementing with any protein powder, always follow the usage recommendations explained on the label.

Finally, when purchasing protein supplements, try to find brands from well-known manufacturers. Avoid obscure, off-brand products or products from unknown international sources. There's very little regulation of the nutritional supplements industry. Products from unknown or nonestablished companies may have poor quality control and may not contain what is stated on the label. Lack of regulatory inspection can also lead to product contamination. These problems are less likely in products manufactured by recognized and well-established food supplement and pharmaceutical companies.

PART SIX

THROUGH THICK AND THIN: WEIGHT CONTROL MADE EASY

CHAPTER 17

Do You Need to Lose Weight?

Ideal Weight versus Healthy Weight

Do you dream of an "ideal" weight—a number on a chart, a figure in your head, the pounds you weighed in high school? Too often we base our ideal weight on what we see in the media—super-sleek fashion models or well-chiseled men. We think we should weigh what they weigh—and look the way they look. That's a dangerous perception, leading to obsessive, unhealthy concerns over weight and appearance. In reality, no specific ideal weight can be assigned to any one individual. What you should weigh depends on many different factors, including height, activity level, diet, sex, genetics, and daily energy needs. Rather than obsess over reaching an ideal weight, it's better to shoot for a *healthy body weight* and a *healthy body composition*. With both, you look good, feel great, and perform better. More important, you're at a much lower risk for heart disease, stroke, diabetes, hypertension, and other weight-related problems.

The following section describes several methods for determining healthy body weight and healthy body composition. Choose the ones that feel most comfortable to you. Some people really need to watch a scale. If you do, select another method that will show you body shape changes as well. By choosing methods that measure different things, you will have the greatest chance to get a truer picture of what high-performance living can do for your body.

Finding Your Healthy Weight

So what should your healthy body weight be? There are a couple of ways to find out. One is a simple calculation designed to identify desirable weight ranges: For men, take 106 lb. for the first 5 ft. of your height, and add 6 lb. for each additional inch to arrive at the midpoint of a healthy weight range. For women, take 100 lb. for the first 5 ft. of your height, and add 5 lb. for each extra inch to get the midpoint of your healthy body weight range.

If you fall within 10 percent on either side (lower or higher) of that midpoint, you're within a healthy weight range. The lower end of the ranges are for small-boned individuals; the upper end, for larger-boned people. To make it easy for you, I've provided healthy weight ranges (with midpoints in bold) in table 17-1.

Table 17-1

HEALTHY WEIGHT RANGES

Height	Women	Men
4' 10"	81–**90**–99	85–**94**–103
4' 11"	86–**95**–105	90–**100**–110
5'	90–**100**–110	95–**106**–117
5' 1"	95–**105**–116	101–**112**–123
5' 2"	99–**110**–121	106–**118**–130
5' 3"	104–**115**–127	112–**124**–136
5' 4"	108–**120**–132	117–**130**–143
5' 5"	113–**125**–138	122–**136**–150
5' 6"	117–**130**–143	128–**142**–156
5' 7"	122–**135**–149	133–**148**–163
5' 8"	126–**140**–154	139–**154**–169
5' 9"	131–**145**–160	144–**160**–176
5' 10"	135–**150**–165	149–**166**–183
5' 11"	140–**155**–171	155–**172**–189
6'	144–**160**–176	160–**178**–196
6' 1"	149–**165**–182	166–**184**–202
6' 2"	153–**170**–187	171–**190**–209
6' 3"	158–**175**–193	176–**196**–216
6' 4"	162–**180**–198	182–**202**–222
6' 5"	167–**185**–204	187–**208**–229
6' 6"	171–**190**–209	193–**214**–235
6' 7"	176–**195**–215	198–**220**–242
6' 8"	180–**200**–220	203–**226**–249
6' 9"	—	209–**232**–255
6' 10"	—	214–**238**–262

Compare your present weight with the ranges on the healthy weight chart. If you're within a healthy weight range, congratulations. But if you're more than 10 percent under the lower end of your range, you may be underweight. Ten percent over the upper end of your range is considered overweight; 20 percent over that upper end may indicate obesity.

As an illustration, suppose you're a man who is 5 ft. 11 in. tall. Your healthy body weight should be around 172 (106 lb. + 66 lb.). But your actual weight is 200—or 28 lb. too heavy. That's about 14 percent (28 lb. divided by 200) over your healthy body weight and can be considered overweight.

Body Mass Index (BMI)

Another measuring method is Body Mass Index (BMI), a ratio of height to weight. It's figured by a mathematical formula: Divide your weight in pounds by your height in inches squared. Then multiply the resulting quotient by 705. A BMI of 25 to 30 is considered overweight, and a BMI above 30 indicates obesity. Using the preceding example again: 200 lb. divided by $(5' 11'')^2$ times 705 equals 28. You'd be in the overweight category by BMI as well.

Weight versus Body Fat

Calculating healthy body weight ranges and figuring out your BMI don't tell the whole story. You need to know how much of your weight is body fat. In the last example, that extra 14 percent of weight could be muscle gained through strength training—a great position to be in. So you see: Overweight doesn't necessarily mean excess fat. It could be muscle. If you're muscular, you might weigh more than what the BMI or healthy weight formula suggests.

Overfat is another matter. It means extra pounds are fat, not muscle. A quick way to see whether you're overfat is to pinch the skin two inches above your belly button. If you can pinch more than one inch of skin in that area, you may be overfat.

Finding Your Body Fat Percentage

To set better fitness goals, it helps to know what's optimal in terms of body fat. Healthy ranges of body fat are 22 to 25 percent for women and 15 to 20 percent for men. If you're an athlete, it might be desirable to have slightly lower percentages. Technically, you're considered overfat if your body fat percentage exceeds 20 percent for men and 25 percent for women.

Unfortunately, there's no simple calculation to figure out your fat pounds. A variety of methods can be used to measure and track body composition. The two methods I recommend are skinfold calipers and body circumference measurements.

Skinfold Calipers

With skinfold calipers, a trained technician pinches the skin at certain sites on the body using a spring-loaded device, which gives measurements in millimeters. As you gain lean tissue and lose body fat through strength training, you should notice body fat reductions in the millimeter readings at each site. Some skinfold tests combine these readings to come up with a total percentage of body fat. This calculation, however, doesn't always give an accurate picture of true changes in body composition or body fat distribution.

Body Circum- ference Measure- ment

This is my preferred method for tracking body changes. Body circumference measurement involves periodically measuring the circularity of your upper arm, chest, waist, hips, thighs, and calves with a tape measure to note changes in size. Using a tape measure, simply measure the circumference of your upper arm, chest, waist, hips, thighs, and calves. Then record these readings. It is more accurate to have someone else do the measurements, rather than doing them on yourself.

Do this every four to six weeks, being careful to position the tape measure in the same place each time you measure a body part. You can even plot your measurements over time as evidence of the positive changes strength training makes in your body.

The Risks of Obesity

Regardless of what method you use, the key is to control your weight before it becomes a problem. Currently, 25 percent of all American adults are obese. Obesity is a risk factor for heart disease, stroke, high blood pressure, diabetes, and some cancers. Other health consequences of obesity include kidney disease, cirrhosis of the liver, and arthritis.

A recent verification of the dangers of gaining body fat comes from Iowa, where a major study made some startling discoveries regarding fat distribution on the body and the risk of death. During a five-year period, researchers examined the health, lifestyle, and mortality information of 41,837 Iowa women who were between the ages of fifty-five and sixty-nine years old. Of the 1,504 deaths reported during the study period, more than 80 percent were related to cancer or heart disease. The risk of death was more than twice as high among those women who had the greatest percentage of upper body fat. The researchers suggested that by altering your fat distribution favorably through diet and exercise, you can lower your risk of dying from these diseases.

If you're obese, your longevity is in jeopardy. Staying active and healthy is definitely contingent on maintaining both a healthy body weight and a healthy body fat percentage.

Determining the Number of Calories You Need to Lose Weight

To a certain extent, losing weight and staying in shape depends on "energy balance," a kind of deposit/withdrawal system your body uses to maintain its weight. You deposit energy in the form of calories and then withdraw, or spend, that energy to live, breathe, move, and exercise. As long as your deposits equal your expenditures, your body generally maintains its weight.

In some cases, if you deposit more calories than your body can spend, you're at risk of gaining weight. Eat fewer calories than you spend, and you'll lose weight. Both conditions describe an energy imbalance, in which the scales are tipped in favor of weight loss or weight gain.

To lose a pound of body fat, you have to create a 3,500-calorie deficit, either by eating less, exercising more, or both. By cutting your total calorie intake by 500 calories each day, for example, you should be able to lose one pound a week (500 calories × 7 days)—a safe rate of weight loss. If you add exercise to this equation and burn any extra calories, your weight loss will be even greater. For more information on how to do that, see chapter 21.

Here's how to determine the calories you'll need each day to reach your weight loss goal (or maintain your weight if you're already at a healthy body weight):

Step 1: Take your healthy body weight (as determined by the weight range formula explained at the beginning of this chapter) and multiply it by 10. This number is the amount of calories you need daily to maintain your heartbeat, breathe, and regulate other basal metabolic functions.

Step 2: Select an activity factor from table 17-2 that corresponds to your activity level. Multiply that factor by your healthy body weight.

Table 17-2

ACTIVITY FACTORS FOR DETERMINING ENERGY NEEDS

Sedentary	Moderately Active	Active	Very Active	Extremely Active
3	4	5	7	10

- *Sedentary:* No exercise, gardening, or housework.
- *Moderately active:* You exercise, garden, do housework three to five times a week for 20 to 30 minutes each time. Also, you use stairs and walk briskly.
- *Active:* You exercise three to five times a week for 60 minutes each session, as well as use stairs and walk briskly.
- *Very Active:* You exercise three to five times a week for 90-plus minutes each session. Or you do more than one 60-minute workout session a day. Also, you use stairs and walk briskly. You may have other daily physical activity as well. Competitive recreational athletes often fit into this category.
- *Extremely Active:* You exercise five or more times a week for 120-plus minutes each session. Or you work out more than 90 minutes a day. You use stairs and walk briskly. Professional athletes often fit into this category.

Step 3: Add the numbers from steps 1 and 2 to arrive at the number of calories you need to eat to lose weight, or to maintain weight if you are already at a healthy body weight.

As an illustration: Suppose you're a woman whose healthy body weight should be 125 pounds, and you're moderately active. Here's how to figure your daily calories for weight loss:

Step 1: $125 \times 10 = 1,250$

Step 2: $125 \times 4 = 500$

Step 3: $1,250 + 500 = 1,750$

Based on this formula, your prescribed caloric level of 1,750 should result in weight loss or maintainence if you're already at your healthy body weight of 125.

Using the High-Performance Menu Plans

The next step is to plan what you're going eat. To help you, use the High-Performance Menu Plans in appendix A. One plan is set up for 1,800 calories a day; the other, for 3,000 calories. These can be adjusted for the caloric level you need for weight loss. If you need to reduce your calories, simply decrease your portions of some foods. But maintain the same ratio of nutrients: 65 percent of your calories should come from complex carbohydrates, 15 percent from protein, and 20 percent from fat. To make sure you're getting all the nutrients you need—and in the right proportions—consult a good calorie-counter book such as *Bowes' and Church's Food*

Values of Portions Commonly Used, 16th edition, by Jean A. T. Pennington (Lippincott-Raven). You should be able to get it from the library or bookstore.

Your diet should be as low in fat as possible, since reducing dietary fat is one of the best ways to shed body fat. By keeping your total fat intake to 20 percent of total daily calories, you may be able to lose body fat with little or no restriction in total calories. Table 17-3 translates this recommendation into actual fat gram intakes for various caloric needs.

Body fat burns in the torch of carbohydrate, so the best weight loss diet is high in carbs. Emphasize vegetables, fruits, breads, cereals, grains, and pastas in your diet. Plus, carbs are the fuel of choice for physical exertion. They burn more efficiently than either protein or fat and will keep your energy level high for your workouts.

As for protein, choose fish, skinless chicken and turkey, and lean red meat like sirloin or round cuts. Stay away from fried and sautéed foods, and eat more steamed, broiled, grilled, baked, and boiled foods.

Be sure to drink plenty of fluids, especially water, to keep your metabolism running clean. Don't skip meals, either. Skipping meals only fools your body into thinking it's starving. It will start to conserve calories rather than burn them, even over a short period of twelve to fifteen hours.

Finally, try to spread your calories out evenly during the day instead of eating a tiny breakfast, a tiny lunch, and a huge dinner. It's best to eat a hearty breakfast. Depending on your appetite, make your lunch large enough to get you through until dinner, or split it up into a small lunch and an afternoon snack. In fact, most people feel best when they eat five to six small meals a day instead of three large meals.

Table 17-3

FAT GRAMS IN A DIET OF 20% TO 25% OF CALORIES AS FAT

Calories per Day	Grams of Fat per Day
1,200	27–33
1,400	31–39
1,600	36–44
1,800	40–50
2,000	44–56
2,200	49–61
2,400	53–67
3,000	60–75

Dinner should always be a lighter meal, especially if you like to snack in the evening. Evening snackers should stick to foods like air-popped popcorn, nonfat frozen yogurt, nonfat milk, fresh fruit, or fresh vegetables. Stay away from fat, especially at night when it's hard to burn off.

Breaking Plateaus

During the early stages of your fat-loss diet, you'll drop weight rapidly, perhaps as much as 5 lb. in the first week. Keep in mind that most of this weight is a loss of water and carbohydrate. When you eat less, your body starts burning up its stored fuel (carbohydrate and fat) for energy. At first most of the fuel used is carbohydrate, stored in the liver and muscle as glycogen. Stored with glycogen is water. In fact, for every part of stored glycogen, there are three parts of water. Suppose your body burns up 400 g of glycogen. Along with the glycogen goes its accompanying water—1,200 g of it. That's a total of 1,600 g or about 3.5 lb. of weight. You can see why so much of your initial weight loss is water. In the first few days of a diet, as much as 70 percent of the weight lost is water.

As you stay on your diet, less of the weight loss will be water and glycogen, and more will be body fat. But a time will come when your rate of loss will slow to a snail's pace, or you'll reach a plateau in which you're no longer losing weight at your prescribed caloric level. This happens because your body requires less energy at a lighter weight. As you trim down, you need fewer calories each day to stay at your new weight.

To break this frustrating sticking point, adjust your calories for further weight loss. The best way to do this is by increasing your activity so that you're using up 250 to 500 more calories a day. Another way to jump-start your weight loss is by reducing your calories by 250 and simultaneously increasing your exercise expenditure by 250 calories. Consult the Energy Expenditure Chart in chapter 21 for calorie-burning activities to help you.

Some Cautions about Calories

Watch your calorie cutting, however. Although it is a calorie deficit that brings about weight loss, calorie cutting can also keep you from losing fat because of the effect it has on your metabolism. In many cases, you'll have to increase your calories for successful weight control. You'll see why in the next chapter.

CHAPTER 18

Successful Weight Control

Beyond Calories

Losing weight is influenced by more than just calories in/calories out. Other factors come into play, including your resting metabolic rate, the composition of your diet, and the amount of exercise you get. Let's take a closer look at these factors, and I think you'll get some excellent insight into what it takes to successfully control your weight. Exercise plays such a critical role in weight loss and control that I've covered it separately in chapter 21.

Your Resting Metabolic Rate (RMR)

The energy it takes to keep your heart beating, your lungs breathing, and other physiological systems working is known as your basal metabolic rate (BMR). It is measured after a person has not moved or eaten for at least twelve hours. Your resting metabolic rate (RMR) includes the BMR plus the additional energy required for being not just awake but alert and sitting up. Your RMR accounts for about 60 to 75 percent of the energy you expend daily.

The higher this rate, the more likely you are to lose fat or maintain a healthy body weight. In a four-year study of Native Americans living in the Southwest, researchers found that individuals with the slowest RMRs gained an average of 6 lb. a year. On average, those with higher RMRs gained only a half a pound a year; some lost less than a pound.

Your resting metabolic rate is closely linked to how much lean muscle you have. The more muscle you have, the higher your RMR. Sex, age, heredity, and physical activity are all factors affecting muscular body composition. Men typically have more muscle than women. Older people have less muscle, since muscles tend to whither as we age. Some people are simply born with a greater percentage of muscle than others. Regardless, you can up your percentage of lean muscle by strength training and following a good nutrition program.

The Starvation Adaptation Response

If cutting calories, never go below 1,200 calories if you're a woman and 1,600 if you're a man. Long periods of calorie deprivation—that is, diets under 1,200 calories a day—lower your RMR as a result of something called the *starvation adaptation response*. This simply means that your metabolism has slowed down to accommodate your lower caloric intake. Your body is stockpiling dietary fat and calories rather than burning them for energy. You can actually gain body fat on a diet of 1,200 calories or less a day.

The starvation adaptation response was first recognized during World War II in the Warsaw ghetto in Poland. People imprisoned there subsisted on very little food, yet they survived much longer than estimated by ghetto physicians. The reason was that their metabolisms had slacked off to allow the body to live and survive. Starvation adaptation is a built-in safety valve—a quite clever one actually—to help us survive.

Adding Calories

If someone isn't losing weight on a reduced-calorie diet, I often advise adding calories. A good illustration is Marla R., a sportswriter. Marla was thirty-eight, 5 ft. 9, and weighed 165 lb. with a body fat level of about 25 percent (slightly high for a woman). Her goal was to lose 10 to 15 lb. and become more fit. At the time I began working with her, she was eating 1,200 calories a day and working out two hours, five times a week.

You'd think with that kind of diet and exercise regimen, she'd be trim and toned to a tee. But she wasn't. In fact, she had been steadily *gaining* weight over the past three years. Either she had underestimated her daily calorie intake, or her body had gone into starvation adaptation. I suspected the latter, which would better account for the weight gain. So I increased her caloric intake just slightly—to 1,500 calories a day to boost her resting metabolic rate back up. This allowed for an average weight loss of 1 to 1.5 lb. a week, the ideal rate for losing weight and maintaining the loss. Marla was highly motivated. She kept up her workouts, stuck to the diet, and was able to drop 10 lb. of mostly body fat over a period of several months.

If you've been dieting at a caloric level of under 1,500 calories a day, plus exercising, without losing body fat, then adjust your calories upward slightly—by 100, 200, or 300 calories a day. Be sure those calories are from carbs, not from fat. This adjustment should prime your metabolism for better weight loss.

Dangers of Very-Low-Calorie Diets

When your calories dip very low—say they drop below 1,200 a day and stay there—you'll really struggle to shed pounds. Not only that, you're putting your health at risk. Diets with insufficient calories don't supply your body with enough nutrients for good health. That spells trouble. Take the case of Al "Bubba" Baker, a former lineman with the Browns. Toward the end of his football career, he was approached by a well-known weight loss company to lose weight quickly as part of a promotional campaign. During spring training, Al went on the diet and was eating around 800 calories a day—in addition to working out twice a day in the hot sun. One day, he passed out on the field and became very ill. He did lose the weight but later regained it. As many people do, he tried the diet again, dropped the weight, but put it right back on. That's when he ended up on my doorstep.

Al had a couple of goals. The first was to trim down, particularly because he was appearing on television as a sports commentator. Second, he wanted a diet that would stave off heart disease. So many of his buddies, ex–football players, had already had coronary bypasses—the offshoot of eating massive amounts of fatty foods during their football years.

I designed a nutrient-rich diet for him, one that fit his lifestyle and would be heart healthy. The weight started peeling off slowly, as planned. Then Al had an offer from national television, and he wanted to accelerate his weight loss. He went back on the weight loss company's program. Once again, he passed out—this time during a live radio broadcast. On the news that night, he blamed the quick weight loss program for his fainting spell. Scared, he vowed to diet the healthy way from then on. As far as I know, he's kept his promise.

When Athletes Diet

The reason most athletes try to trim body fat is to improve their performance. A lot of athletes, however, are walking a thin line when it comes to calories. A case in point is Joanne B., a swim coach in her early forties who competes in Masters swim competition. Even though she was very lean (13 percent body fat) at 5 ft. 10 and 150 lb., she wanted to lose a little weight to become lighter for competition, so she cut her calories. The trouble was, however, that Joanne started feeling tired all the time. After reviewing a three-day diet record she filled out for me, I found she was eating 2,862 calories a day, with 16 percent of the calories coming from protein, 57 percent from carbs, and 27 percent from fat.

I could see the problem right away. Joanne had cut her calories just enough that she was slowing down in her workouts and didn't have enough energy to perform other daily activities. What's more, she hadn't lost any weight with this approach, most likely because her resting metabolic rate had plunged. Had she continued this way, she would have started to lose muscle and gain body fat.

I increased her calories to between 3,000 and 3,500 a day. Plus, I adjusted her carbs upward to 60 percent and her fat downward to 24 percent. This made a huge difference. Joanne became stronger in her workouts and felt much better overall. Ultimately, she broke into the World Top Ten rankings in the 400 I.M. event and was ranked in the National Top Ten thirteen times in 1994.

The point is, low-calorie diets are a disaster for anyone wanting to maintain or build muscle. Such diets can lower your RMR and cause your body to burn healthy muscle and store unsightly fat. You often have to push calories upward slightly to get the results you want.

The Role of Diet Composition in Losing Weight

After you eat a meal, your metabolic rate goes up as food is digested and metabolized. Technically this is known as the *thermic effect of food* (TEF) and makes up about 10 percent of the energy you expend each day. As with your resting metabolic rate, eating more calories increases the thermic effect of food—another reason not to cut calories too low.

Why Fat Calories Turn to Body Fat

In addition to calorie burning, one of the most significant factors influencing the thermic effect of food is the composition of the food you eat—that is, the proportion of carbohydrate, protein, and fat on your plate. The biggest concern is fat. Eating too much fat promotes fat storage. The fat you eat turns into fat on your body much more easily than carbohydrate and protein do.

One animal study I like to cite involves two groups of rats, both eating equivalent calorie diets. One diet was high in carbs and low in fat; the other, higher in fat. The rats on the high-carbohydrate diet maintained their weight and their percentage of body fat, whereas the rats on the high-fat diet became obese—20 percent fatter than the other group.

Similar results—that all calories are not created equal—have been shown in people. One study compared the fat intake of 205 adult women with their body fat percentages as measured by skinfold calipers. The researchers had the women fill out questionnaires about their diets and various lifestyle factors, including exercise. The data showed that the most significant predictor of fatness was fat in the diet. Fat calories are more likely to be deposited as body fat.

The reason is that very little energy is expended to process fat, compared with carbohydrates. The energy cost (TEF) of metabolizing carbs and converting them to glycogen for storage is rated at 25 percent, in contrast to just 4 percent to store fat. In other words, your body works harder at breaking down carbs and using them for energy. Not so with fat. The body recognizes fat as fat and prefers to hang on to it rather than break it down for energy.

How Sugar Produces Body Fat

Fat in the diet isn't the only villain affecting body fat. Sugar is to blame, too, which is why I recommend cutting out sugar-laced foods if you're trying to pare down. Not long ago, researchers at Indiana University analyzed the diets of four groups of people: lean men (average body fat was 15 percent); lean women (average body fat was 20 percent); obese men (average body fat was 25 percent); and obese women (average body fat was 35 percent).

The obese men and women ate more of their calories from fat (as high as 36 percent of total calories) and refined sugars such as candy, doughnuts, and ice cream, which are also high in fat. Also, too much refined sugar can cause the body to overproduce the hormone insulin, a reaction that stimulates fat production. In addition, the obese subjects didn't eat very much fiber compared with the groups of lean men and women.

Cutting Down on Fat and Sugary Foods

The lesson here: Change the composition of your diet to better manage your weight. This means cutting down on fat and sugary foods. The easiest way to do this is by increasing the complex carbs in your diet. Remember, 65 percent of your total daily calories should come from carbs—more if you strength-train.

High-carb foods happen to be fiber-smart choices too. Fiber keeps calories moving through your system faster, plus makes you feel full. A healthy weight loss diet includes lots of high-fiber foods from complex carbohydrates. Shoot for a goal of 25 to 35 g of fiber daily.

As for sugary foods, limit them in your fat-loss program. Instead, make a beeline to natural complex carbs like whole grains, rice, legumes, potatoes, and vegetables. By eating more of these foods, you'll automatically cut your fat intake, plus increase your vitamins and minerals. Your body will thank you for it too, since it prefers to burn up carbs for energy rather than store them as fat.

You must also cut down on fats, which isn't as hard as you might think. By concentrating on high-carb eating, you naturally end up eating smaller portions of fat.

Drastic Changes Aren't Necessary

As you begin to modify your diet for fat loss, don't make drastic changes. They just don't work, especially over the long term. While I was working with the Cleveland Browns, we decided to take out all fat from the players' menus at training camp. No more fried chicken, fried fish, or french fries.

The initial menus I designed included some lightly fried chicken and fish twice a week. Having these foods once in a while certainly wasn't going to hurt guys weighing around 225 lb. with only 15 percent body fat. But after some deliberation, we took a harder line. Out went all the fat.

About three weeks into the five-week training camp, there was a mutiny. The players were furious over the menus, and they directed their anger toward me. They refused to eat the food. In desperation, I solicited their suggestions on what they wanted to eat, and fried chicken was voted back in. So we put fried chicken back on the menu, but it was one of four entrées the players could select—and the only fried food.

The moral of this story is that dietary changes should not be made all at once. By putting so much pressure on yourself, you only set yourself up for failure. Make changes slowly and keep your sights on your ultimate goal: a trim, healthier, more active body.

CHAPTER 19

Lifestyle Diet Planning

No-Sacrifice Nutrition

Dieting doesn't mean giving up your favorite foods. It's still possible to have your cake and eat it, too. Simply moderate how much of your favorite foods you eat by having them less often, and then learn how to make healthier substitutions.

One of my greatest nutritional challenges in this regard was a rookie football player for the Cleveland Browns who wanted to lose weight to improve his speed on the field. Unless he trimmed down, his chance to be on the team was in jeopardy, so we needed a dramatic nutritional rescue.

At the time I started working with him, he was eating slightly over 7,000 calories a day. Broken down, those calories figured out to 17 percent protein, 32 percent fat, and about 49 percent carbohydrate. In daily fat grams, he was consuming a whopping 250 a day. Based on his goals, I overhauled his diet down to 5,680 calories a day—with 12.5 percent of those calories coming from protein, 25 percent from fat, and 62.5 percent from carbs. That mix would slash his fat grams to a healthier 142 g a day.

But this was no easy task. Like most rookies, this athlete lived in a hotel and ate all his meals at restaurants. Portion control wasn't a problem, but hidden fat was. There was so much fat lurking in his food that we had to take some drastic measures. Take milk, for example. He was gulping down close to a half a gallon of 2 percent milk a day. That added up to a lot of fat! Time for a change. I recommended that he switch to 1 percent or skim milk and replace some of the milk with ice tea or fruit juices.

Dinner for him was often fried chicken, another habit that had to be moderated. In its place, we substituted skinless broiled chicken, drizzled with barbecue sauce for flavor. Also, I suggested that he load up on complex carbs like rice, pasta, bread, and vegetables and cut his meat allotment down to about 8 oz. a day.

Most of the time he ate at a small mom-and-pop restaurant that specialized in home cooking. The owners were more than happy to work with us on his diet. After all, he was a big guy who ate a lot, so they could always make a separate pot of food just for him. Instead of the usual greens laced with pork fat, they flavored the vegetables with onion, garlic, vinegar, and beef bouillon, along with some lean ham for taste. There was one dish he didn't want to give up—sweet potato pie. He didn't have to. We simply modified the original recipe, substituting skim milk for evaporated milk, diet margarine for butter, and one egg yolk for every two whites. The modified pie was delicious. Ultimately we worked out an entire game plan for eating out at restaurants without sabotaging his diet.

The upshot of all this was that he lost the weight, made the team, and had a great season. He's now playing for another NFL team and has always credited some of his success to the dietary changes he made.

Building in Your Favorite Foods

When I plan diets for my clients, I always build their favorite foods into the program. Remember Marla R., the sports reporter described in the previous chapter? If you recall, she was having trouble losing weight, most likely because her body was in a starvation adaptation mode due to low-calorie dieting. I made a slight adjustment in her diet so that she was eating more calories a day (1,500), with a better distribution of proteins, carbs, and fat.

Marla attended a lot of work-related social events. That being the case, she didn't want to compromise her lifestyle to exclude herself from parties she enjoyed. The big question for Marla was what to do about drinking alcohol. No problem. We agreed that it was fine for her to include a glass (3.5 oz.) of wine a day in her diet plan. On days when she might drink more, she needed to plan ahead and adjust her diet. Marla did this by removing two fat servings for each serving of alcohol, either 3.5 oz. of wine, 12 oz. of light beer, or 1 oz. of hard liquor.

I recommended that she not overdo this, however. When there's alcohol in the system, the liver starts working overtime to metabolize it and can't concentrate on fat-burning. Too much alcohol would compromise her fat loss. Not only that, it jeopardizes the body's use of vitamins and minerals. The one-glass-a-day rule could stick, but drinking more than that on a frequent basis would be risky.

Adjusting for Splurges

Let's face it: Every now and then, you want to splurge on treats not on your plan. Don't worry—you can, and still achieve your goal. A good example is Gail F., a thirty-eight-year-old modern dancer and dance instructor. Gail indulged herself in occasional splurges such as pizza and desserts. This is perfectly all right, as long as you adjust for your "splurge" calories. In Gail's case, I advised that she eat a lower-fat, high-carbohydrate lunch whenever she planned to eat a high-fat dinner. That way, the entire day wouldn't be lopsided in favor of fat. You can do the same. Suppose you're having dinner at a restaurant and want some dietary leeway. Simply eat lightly and in a low-fat manner earlier in the day.

A word of caution though: If you've grown accustomed to high-carb, low-fat eating, and you have a high-fat meal for dinner, you may not feel so good the next day. Thanks to better dietary habits, your body is no longer used to digesting a lot of fat, and you could get diarrhea or cramps.

Gail also liked desserts, so I planned her diet accordingly. Most days during the week, she'd eat fruit for dessert. While fulfilling her desire for something sweet after dinner, this plan solved a couple of other nutritional problems. First, it boosted her fiber intake. At the time we met, Gail was eating a mere 4.5 g of fiber a day (25 to 35 g are recommended). Plus, it upped her carb intake, which had been too low (52 percent of total calories) for her activity level and occupation.

Strategies for Eating "Forbidden Foods"

When I worked in the preventive cardiology program at Duke University, one of my responsibilities was to develop healthy recipes for people in the South, who traditionally eat a lot of high-fat fare and have higher rates of heart disease as a result. Through that experience I discovered that many fat-laced recipes can be converted into healthy low-fat versions without sacrificing taste.

With the right planning, any food can fit into a fat-loss diet, and nearly any recipe can be adapted to low-fat fare. So instead of thinking you can never eat any of your favorite foods again, make some minor changes in recipes and then enjoy them to your heart's content. Here are several strategies to help you:

- Be sure to trim the fat from any meat before cooking. The skin from poultry can be removed after cooking. Then brown meats by broiling, grilling, or cooking in nonstick pans with little or no oil. For beef, select the "skinniest six" listed in chapter 8: eye of round, round tip, top round, top loin, tenderloin, and sirloin. The "select" cut is always leanest.
- When making soups, stews, sauces, and broths, you can remove 100 calories of fat per tablespoon by chilling the liquid after cooking and skimming off the congealed fat.
- Use fresh fruit whenever possible. When using canned products such as fish or fruits, purchase those packed in water rather than oil or heavy syrup.
- In recipes for baked products, the sugar can often be reduced ¼ to ⅓ without harming the final product. Cinnamon and vanilla also lend sweetness.
- For sauces and dressings, use low-calorie bases such as vinegar, mustard, tomato juice, and fat-free bouillon, instead of high-calorie ones like cream, fats, oils, and mayonnaise.

Table 19-1

TO CUT SATURATED FAT

Use	Instead of
Soft vegetable margarines and oils	Butter, lard, bacon, and chicken fat
Nonfat yogurt or light sour cream	Sour cream
Skim milk	Whole milk
Low-fat cheeses	Whole milk cheeses
Egg whites or egg substitutes	Whole eggs

Note: Many cheeses, although made with skim milk, have cream added to them. Check labels for fat content.

Table 19-2

RECIPE SUBSTITUTIONS

Use	Instead of
⅞ cup vegetable oil, 1 cup tub margarine*	1 cup of butter
Equal part of applesauce	Fat or oil in quick breads and other baked goods
1 cup evaporated skimmed milk	1 cup heavy cream
¼ cup egg substitute**	1 medium whole egg
1 cup skim milk yogurt	1 cup high-fat yogurt (plain)
1 cup light sour cream or 1 cup skim milk yogurt	1 cup sour cream
3 tbsp. cocoa powder, plus 1 tbsp. vegetable oil	1 oz. baking chocolate

Note: The first ingredient in margarines should be a liquid polyunsaturated oil.

**Some egg substitutes do contain cholesterol. Check label to be sure.

- Substitute the fat or oil with an equal amount of applesauce in baked products. Applesauce is a wonderful replacement for the fat in baked products such as quick breads.
- Cut the saturated fat, without sacrificing flavor, by making smart low-fat substitutes as shown in the tables 19-1 and 19-2.

Dining Out

If you're like a lot of people, you want to get out of the kitchen occasionally and let someone else do the cooking for you. But what about your diet? Does dining out spell diet disaster? Not necessarily. You can take control of your menu and your meal at restaurants. The trick is to have a game plan before you go.

To start with, choose a restaurant that serves nutritious, low-fat choices: chicken, fish, salads, baked potatoes, steamed vegetables, to name just a few. Avoid all-you-can-eat buffets and restaurants that only offer high-calorie, low-nutrient items. If you know you'll be dining out one evening, eat lighter during the day. That way you can have some leeway at dinner. Before arriving at the restaurant, decide what you'll order, and how you'd like it prepared—chicken without the skin, baked or grilled fish, lean red meat, or a vegetarian entrée, for example.

Beware of fat hiding in certain restaurant foods. Sauces, condiments, butter, oil, mayonnaise, creams, and rich cheeses all add a lot of fat to appetizers, entrées, and side dishes. Ask the serving staff to leave out high-fat ingredients. Another option is to make a substitution, such as a baked potato for french fries.

Request that sauces, salad dressings, and sour cream be served on the side so you can control the amount that you use. Request that a menu item be prepared using an alternative method, such as broiling instead of frying.

Be inquisitive! Ask questions about foods on the menu. Be specific! How is the food prepared? What are the ingredients? To help you, consult the following "menu dictionary" (see table 19-3), which shows what to choose and what to avoid.

Mexican Restaurants

With all the bad press Mexican restaurants have gotten over their high-fat fare, I've had a lot of clients asking about whether they should eat at these establishments. The basic ingredients of Mexican-style dishes are generally low-fat, high-carbohydrate foods like beans, rice, tortillas, fresh vegetables, and fresh fruit. Fish and chicken are the typical protein dishes. But many restaurants prepare these foods by frying or adding lots of cheese and sour cream. This only negates their health value.

You can still enjoy Mexican foods without the fat guilt. At a restaurant, skip the fried tortilla chips and nachos. They're high in fat and salt. Instead, order plain baked tortillas to dip in your salsa. Try light and low-fat gazpacho soup for your appetizer. Good alternatives to fried foods are grilled foods, such as fajitas, mesquite grilled chicken or fish, or baked entrées.

Check with the server to see whether the refried beans are prepared in lard or baked or boiled, and seasoned. If they aren't refried, enjoy them. They make great high-carb foods. Rice is usually safe, but find out whether fat is added, just in case.

Watch out for guacamole! Contrary to most other fruits, avocados—the basic ingredient of guacamole—are as high in fat as butter. Ask that guacamole, cheese, and sour cream toppings be served on the side. That way you can control how much you'll be eating.

You can make your own nachos at home by baking tortillas until crisp, or using new products such as baked corn chips, low-fat cheese, and light sour cream. Most vegetarian cookbooks or recently published Mexican cookbooks have recipes for beans that are boiled or baked with seasonings, and not refried. You can even drain a can of beans, mash and season them. Voilà, beans that are great for burritos and enchiladas.

Table 19-3

MENU DICTIONARY

Choose (Low in Fat)	Avoid (High in Fat)
Entrées	*Entrées*
In their own juices	Fried
Boiled	Sautéed
Broiled	Au gratin
Grilled	Buttery, buttered
Baked	Creamed, cream sauce
Roasted	Hollandaise
Poached	Alfredo
Lean meats (round, sirloin, tenderloin, flank steak, filet mignon)	Parmesan
	Marinated (in oil)
Garden fresh	Casserole
Tomato juice	Gravy
	Hash
	Potpie
	Crispy
Appetizers	*Appetizers*
Steamed seafood, including mussels, clams, crabs, lobsters, or shrimp	Swimming in butter
	Cheese
Raw or steamed vegetables	
Vegetable antipasto	
Soups	*Soups*
Gazpacho, consommé, broth-type	Creamed
Vegetables	*Vegetables*
Fresh, raw or steamed	Fried
Baked potato or yams	Heavily buttered, creamed, or in cheese sauce
Salads	*Salads*
With oil and vinegar or other clear dressings	With meats, bacon, cheese, or croutons
With oil-free diet dressings	With creamy dressings

Table 19-3 (continued)

Choose (Low in Fat)	**Avoid (High in Fat)**
Breads	*Breads*
Plain	Baked with butter, shortening, or cheese
Breadsticks	Sweet rolls
Hard rolls	
English muffins	
Sandwiches	*Sandwiches*
Tuna, chicken, turkey, seafood, or lean cooked beef	Processed lunch meats, hard cheese, fried foods
	Sandwiches with sauces, gravies, mayonnaise, or bacon
Desserts	*Desserts*
Fruit, sorbet, sherbet, angel food cake, and other specially made low-fat items	Commercial pies, cakes, yogurt, pastries, ice cream, and candies

Make the most of the new light sour creams and low-fat cheeses, too. Read the labels carefully. Some "lite" cheese may just be low in salt, or low in cholesterol, but not low in fat. Also, learn to use the fresh herb and fruit combinations, like cilantro and lime juice that make Mexican cooking so wonderful. Be creative. You'll find that you'll enjoy discovering new light ways of preparing your favorite dishes.

Fast Food   Remember the NFL football player described earlier? He loved to eat fast food, especially BK Broilers (32 percent fat) and Egg McMuffins. Nonetheless, I didn't ban him from fast-food restaurants. I taught him how to make healthy fast-food choices. For example, rather than eat two BK Broilers, I suggested he eat just one and add a salad instead. For dessert, he had been eating ice cream. I persuaded him to switch to low-fat yogurt. Instead of loading up on Egg McMuffins every morning, he started alternating those between cereal, fruit juice, and milk at McDonald's. When he found out what he could eat, he ended up enjoying fast food even more. You can do the same by making the right selections at fast-food restaurants. See table 19-4 for some guidance in choosing fast foods.

Here are some additional fast-food tips to keep you on track:

- Always order the regular-sized sandwiches; they're lower in fat.
- In place of a bigger sandwich, order a salad, low-fat milk, and low-fat frozen yogurt to complete your meal.
- Stay away from fried foods.

Table 19-4

YOUR BEST FAST-FOOD BETS

	Calories	Percent of Fat
Arby's		
Shakes		
Chocolate	451	23
Jamocha	368	26
Vanilla	330	31
Blueberry muffin	200	25
Cinnamon nut danish	340	25
Chocolate chip cookie	130	28
Plain baked potato	240	7
Chicken fajita pita	272	31
Grilled chicken barbeque	378	34
Lite chicken deluxe	263	21
Lite ham deluxe	255	19
Lite roast beef deluxe	294	31
Lite roast turkey deluxe	260	17
French dip roast beef	345	32
Beef with vegetables and barley soup	96	26
Old-fashioned chicken noodle soup	99	16
Tomato florentine soup	84	16
Burger King		
Shakes		
Chocolate syrup added	409	24
Vanilla syrup added	334	27
Bagel sandwich: ham, egg, and cheese	438	35
Chocolate brownie (Weight Watchers)	100	27
Lemon pie	290	25
Mocha pic (Weight Watchers)	160	28
Frozen yogurt		
Chocolate	132	20
Vanilla	120	23

Table 19-4 (continued)

Burger King (*continued*)	**Calories**	**Percent of Fat**
Angel hair pasta with cheese (Weight Watchers)	210	21
Angel hair pasta without cheese (Weight Watchers)	160	11
BK Broiler sandwich	267	32
Broiled chicken sandwich (no dressing)	140	26
Chunky chicken salad (no dressing)	142	25
Veggie Sticks	60	15
McDonald's		
Low-fat shakes	320	5
Cheerios	80	11
Wheaties	90	10
English muffin with spread	170	21
Hotcakes with margarine and syrup	440	25
McDonaldland cookies	290	28
Soft-serve ice cream	140	29
Chunky chicken salad (no dressing)	150	24
Lite vinaigrette dressing (1 tbsp.)	12	38
Hamburger	255	32
McLean deluxe	320	28
Pizza Hut		
Cheese pizza (2 medium slices)	518	35
Cheese pan pizza (2 medium slices)	492	33
Taco Bell		
Bean burrito	387	33
Chicken burrito	334	32
Combination burrito	407	35
Wendy's		
Apple Danish	360	35
Frosty (12 oz.)	340	26
Chili (small)	190	28
Chili (large)	290	28
Bacon and cheese baked potato	510	30

Table 19-4 (continued)

Wendy's (*continued*)	Calories	Percent of Fat
Broccoli and cheese baked potato	450	28
Plain baked potato	300	2
Caesar side salad	160	34
Grilled chicken sandwich	290	22
Junior hamburger	270	30
Kid's meal hamburger	270	30

- Don't eat the high-fat tortilla shells from taco salads.
- Request that sour cream and secret sauces be left off your order.
- Top your baked potato with chili instead of fatty cheese sauce.
- Whatever you order, order just one!

Pizza Restaurants

Pizza is actually a great fast food, especially if you're active. The crust is high in carbs, the tomato sauce is fat-free, and the cheese is usually made from part-skim milk mozzarella. It's the toppings that can throw you off course. Stick to all veggie pizzas, and don't add extra cheese. If you detect any extra oil floating on the top, dab it off with a napkin before you dig in.

But when it comes to portion control, don't be like baseball's great Yogi Berra, who, after ordering a pizza, was asked whether he wanted it cut into four or eight pieces. "Better make it four," he replied. "I don't think I can eat eight."

Please don't eat the whole pizza! Have just two slices, complemented by a salad, and share the rest with friends.

Holiday Eating

If you're interested in sticking to a healthful diet and regular exercise routine, the season of celebration can be frustrating. Attending countless office parties, cocktail receptions, and dinner celebrations "weighs heavily" on your body and mind. What's more, taking time out for gift shopping and entertainment preparation often infringes upon precious exercise time. These short but intense lifestyle interruptions can make you feel out of sorts, sometimes displacing holiday cheer. But your next holiday season can be different.

The key to a guilt-free holiday is to set realistic goals. If you're trying to shed weight, you may not continue to lose at the same rate during this season. In fact, it may be unreasonable to expect to lose any weight during the holidays. Maintaining your present weight, or only gaining 2 or 3 lb. instead of 8 or 10, is a more sensible goal.

Regardless of what comes between you and your workout, try not to eliminate it all together. If you're like most people, you need to let off some steam during the often stressful holiday season, and exercise is the perfect stress reliever. Plus, it burns off the extra calories you've eaten.

On party days, plan light meals and snacks so you feel free to enjoy richer foods at the event. Eat something small before you go to avoid arriving too hungry. When we're ravenous, our stomachs and eyes make our food choices instead of our brains. Remember that this is probably not the only party you'll be attending, so you don't need to eat everything all at one place to feel like you've celebrated.

It's easy to make food the central focus of holiday celebrations. You arrive at a party and head straight for the table or the bar. We're busy eating and drinking for the entire evening. Why not concentrate on people instead? Get more involved in conversation than in food.

When you do eat, make smart choices. Splurge with fresh fruits and vegetables. Take smaller servings of high-fat dips and rich desserts. You needn't finish everything on your plate, either. Just tasting a little bit of a lot of food may satisfy your palate and your curiosity. At buffets, select a small plate, take only one serving, and carefully arrange the food on your plate instead of piling it up.

Table 19-5

SAMPLE THANKSGIVING DINNER MENU

Holiday Food	Calories
1 gin and tonic or screwdriver	175
Cheese and crackers appetizer	350
Turkey and gravy, 10-oz. portion	200
Stuffing, 1 cup	400
Sweet potato pie, 1 piece	245
Peas and carrots, ½ cup, with butter	90
Corn bread, 2 pieces, with butter	435
Cranberry sauce, ½ cup	210
Wine, two 4-oz. glasses	175
Pumpkin pie with whipped cream, 1 slice	260
Coffee with cream and sugar, 2 cups	75
Total calories	2,615

During the holiday season, alcohol flows plentifully. Alcohol is calorically dense (7 calories per gram, compared with 4 calories per gram for carbohydrate), especially when mixed with sweetened beverages. It also stimulates the appetite. You can avoid drinking alcohol, and still remain social, by drinking juice, seltzers, sodas, or tonic waters with a twist of orange, lemon, or lime. If you drink alcohol, alternate alcoholic beverages with these same nonalcoholic selections. Ounce for ounce, cranberry juice cocktail has 60 percent fewer calories than a gin and tonic, and 15 percent fewer calories than a glass of champagne.

What about holiday dinners? They're enough to throw a nutritious eater into a tizzy. For someone who eats moderately sized portions, the traditional Thanksgiving dinner fare weighs in at about 2,600 calories. If larger portions are eaten, or more butter and fat used in cooking and seasoning the food, the calories only go up from there. Table 19-5 shows how a menu stacks up in calorie content.

If, after all your planning, you do overindulge, don't feel guilty. Guilt only weakens your resolve to maintain healthy habits, not to mention that it spoils the fun of holiday celebrations.

Parties

Having a party? Plan your menu with a variety of foods to allow for healthy choices. Snack foods like popcorn, baked tortilla chips, pretzels, or vegetables with dip are lower in fat and calories than nuts or potato and corn chips.

Create lower-fat foods by altering recipes and using low-fat substitutes for high-fat ingredients. For example, replace all or part of the sour cream in dip recipes with light sour cream or plain low-fat yogurt, and use a light mayonnaise in place of regular mayo. When baking or cooking, use two egg whites in place of each whole egg specified, or use egg substitutes. Some of the high-fat cheeses and creams can be replaced by lower-fat products. Quantities of salt, sugar, and other sweeteners in recipes can often be reduced. If you prefer to serve a fat and calorie-packed food, preparing smaller portions is a healthy alternative.

Let's talk turkey again: Self-basting turkeys are higher in fat than plain turkeys. Use a drip pan when roasting so that meats don't sit in the fatty drippings while cooking.

Also, serve meats au jus instead of with gravy. Chill the juices or add ice to congeal the fat for skimming. A fat separator is a great kitchen gadget. You can also add flour or cornstarch to thicken the fat-free juices to prepare a very low fat gravy.

When preparing onions, celery, and mushrooms for stuffings or casseroles, microwave or simmer them in a small amount of water rather than sautéing in butter or oil. Butter can be eliminated from stuffings completely by using Butter Buds and following the directions included with the product.

Good Nutrition While Traveling

It's hard enough to stick to your diet when at home, let alone while you're traveling. Many familiar habits and conditions are disrupted during travel, especially when traveling cross-country or overseas. Changes in diet, exercise, sleep patterns, noise, and temperature throw you out of kilter, affecting your emotions and behavior. I've often arrived at my destination feeling like the luggage in the cargo hold. But over the years, I've learned that a little planning and preparation can make traveling a much more comfortable experience. Here are some recommendations:

✔ Start your trip well rested but feeling a bit of muscle fatigue so that you won't mind sitting so much. If traveling in the morning, schedule a maximum exercise workout the day before departure. If traveling at night, have a hard workout early that same day.

✔ Begin a light diet twelve hours before departure, and maintain that style of eating throughout most of your trip. It will help you feel more comfortable at the outset of your trip and help avoid some of the dietary hazards of overseas travel.

By light diet I mean breads, cereals, vegetables, fruit, and low-fat dairy products. Fish, poultry, legumes, grains, and small amounts of eggs and cheese are good primary protein sources. Eat small portions of beef and stay away from fat-laden foods such as sauces and creams, fried foods, and rich desserts.

✔ Never travel hungry. It puts you at the mercy of the fast-food snack vendors and the often poorly planned airline meal plans. Take light and healthful snack foods with you, such as fresh or dried fruits, salt-free pretzels, or light cheese and hearty whole grain bread. Many major airports now have food vendors selling fresh and dried fruits, nuts, popcorn, soft pretzels, and low-fat fresh or frozen yogurt. If you're ambitious, bring your own food to eat on the plane. Homemade turkey sandwiches or even a carton of nonfat yogurt and cut-up vegetables are easy to pack in a sack.

✔ Consider requesting the special meals available on most airlines, such as seafood, fruit platters, and vegetarian meals. They're lower in fat and cholesterol than the regular fare. These meals must be requested through your ticket agent at least twenty-four hours in advance.

✔ Drink plenty of liquids. The controlled cabin environment is very dry, and you could become dehydrated. Dehydration causes headaches, constipation, and other complaints. When it's time for refreshments, ask for the entire can of juice, seltzer, or soda, instead of just a glassful. Water, and sometimes bottled water, is always available. The extra fluid may mean more visits to the bathroom, but it will also give you a good reason to get up and stretch during the flight.

✔ Avoid caffeine until the end of your flight. It increases your fluid loss and may lead to dehydration. The same goes for alcohol. If you wish to drink alcohol during a flight, limit yourself to one drink, and order a light one such as a wine spritzer.

✔ Adjust your biological time clock by following the local time schedule immediately. This will help you avoid long-term jet lag. A short nap after arrival is fine, but don't sleep your first day away.

CHAPTER 20

Sugar and Fat Substitutes

Alternatives to Sweets and Fats

Sugar-free and fat-reduced foods have become a way of life for people trying to slim down. Approximately 173 million Americans now consume these products, and their use is on the rise. According to the Calorie Control Council, the number of people eating light food and drinking light beverages grew by 32 million between 1991 and 1994.

Cutting down on fat and sugar is certainly an important move if you're trying to shed excess weight. One way to do that is by using sugar substitutes and fat replacers. These products certainly have a place in nutrition, but a concern of mine is that some people may get so carried away with eating fat- and sugar-free foods that they'll eat even fewer nutrient-dense foods such as fruits, vegetables, and grains. That's risky, since both your performance and health could suffer. Using substitutes in moderation is fine, as long as you don't get carried away. Here's what you need to know about these products to stay on the safe side nutritionally.

Sugar Alcohols

Years ago, when "thin is in" became the motto of our increasingly weight-obsessed society, food companies raced to make products that could satisfy our sweet tooth as well as trim our waistlines. Two types of sugar replacements were born: sugar alcohols and artificial sweeteners.

Related to table sugar (sucrose), sugar alcohols include mannitol, sorbitol, and xylitol. All three contain the same number of calories as sugar (4 calories per gram). So if you're trying to cut calories, sugar alcohols offer little benefit. Mannitol and sorbitol are less sweet than sugar, so more must be used to match the sweetness of sugar. This increases the calories in food even more, compared with using sugar.

Sugar alcohols are more slowly absorbed than sugar is. For this reason, the sugar alcohols are thought to be better than sugar for diabetics, who have trouble metabolizing sugar quickly enough to keep blood sugar at healthy levels. The big plus for sugar alcohols, however, is that they don't promote tooth decay.

It's important to point out that sugar alcohols can cause some unpleasant gastrointestinal side effects, namely bloating, flatulence (gas), and diarrhea. Read product ingredient labels carefully to identify foods made with sugar alcohols. Sucrose is the only legally defined sugar for product labeling. That means any product may be called sugar-free as long as it doesn't have any sucrose in it. A sugar-free product may still contain sugar alcohols, or any other sweetener, such as fructose, honey, or molasses.

Artificial Sweeteners

Artificial sweeteners are no strangers to fitness-minded consumers. Products like saccharin were originally developed to help diabetics and improve the taste of other medically supervised diets. Today lab-created sweeteners have found a much broader market among the weight-conscious. Besides saccharin, other sweeteners include cyclamate, acesulfame-K, and by far the most popular, aspartame. All have passed the scrutinizing eye of the FDA, but not without some ups and downs.

Saccharin and Cyclamate

Artificial sweeteners contain fewer calories than sugar and don't promote tooth decay. Saccharin, a zero-calorie sweetener, has been around since 1900 and is used mostly in soft drinks and secondarily as a tabletop sweetener. Another noncalorie sweetener is cyclamate, introduced in the 1950s. It tasted better than saccharin and became enormously popular as a result. But in 1970, because of claims that cyclamate increased the risk of cancer in animals, the FDA banned its use in foods.

Questions regarding the safety of saccharin surfaced in 1977, when experiments suggested it caused bladder tumors in rats. The FDA wanted to ban saccharin too, but the public outcry was so great that this move was halted. Instead of a ban, a warning label became required for all saccharin-containing foods.

Do these sweeteners really cause cancer? The research data are conflicting and can be interpreted in many different ways. The U.S. and Canadian governments completely disagree on their interpretation of the research. In the United States, for example, cyclamate is banned, and saccharin is legal. In Canada, saccharin is banned, and cyclamate is restricted to use as a tabletop sweetener—but only on the advice of a physician—and as a sweetening agent in medicines.

Aspartame

When aspartame was approved for use in 1981, our health worries about artificial sweeteners were over—or so it seemed. Aspartame is an artificially synthesized compound of two natural ingredients (the amino acids phenylalanine and aspartic acid). It appeared to carry none of the blemished laboratory history borne by its predecessors. Aspartame is a protein containing 4 calories per gram. Virtually calorie-free, it's 200 times sweeter than sugar, so far less is necessary to achieve the same sweetness.

The biggest drawback of aspartame is that it can't be used during cooking. Heating breaks the bond between the two amino acids, and its sweetness is lost. Because aspartame tastes so much like sugar and was assumed to be harmless, in three years it surpassed the sales of saccharin and was available in nearly fifty products.

Shortly after the FDA expanded its list of foods approved for the addition of aspartame, questions about its safety cropped up. It was already known that eating aspartame could be dangerous for people with phenylketonuria (PKU), an inability to metabolize phenylalanine (one of the two amino acids in aspartame). That being so, a warning label was required on all products containing aspartame.

But the potential risks to normal, healthy people cast a shadow of doubt on this miracle sweetener. The Centers for Disease Control and Prevention (CDCP) once received some five hundred individual complaints about side effects associated with aspartame use, ranging from headaches and nausea to more severe neurological problems. Few of these claims were ever substantiated, however. After review, the CDC concluded that some people may have vague, nondangerous symptoms caused by an unusual sensitivity to aspartame.

One case in particular, however, deserves mention. A few years after aspartame was approved, an active twenty-four-year-old woman who had always been weight-conscious returned from the Middle East complaining of head pain. As it worsened, she consulted her doctor, who diagnosed the pain as debilitating migraine and cluster headaches. Her condition gradually got more severe until, after spending eighteen out of twenty-four months in the hospital, the true cause was finally discovered.

Even though aspartame had been available since 1981 in the United States, it wasn't available in the Middle East, so the young woman hadn't been exposed to the sweetener. Upon return to the United States, she started drinking aspartame-sweetened soft drinks daily. As her headaches got worse, she had trouble eating. So she drank even more diet soda. The final diagnosis turned out to be severe aspartame/monosodium glutamate (MSG) sensitivity, complicated by the large doses of drugs she was taking for the headaches. Once the drugs were stopped and the aspartame and MSG were removed, she quickly recovered.

Acesulfame-K

A more recently approved sweetener is acesulfame potassium (or acesulfame-K). Marketed under the name Sunette, acesulfame-K is as sweet as aspartame but more stable and less expensive. Acesulfame-K is approved for use in chewing gum, beverages, instant coffee and tea, gelatins, and puddings. Consumer groups are worried about its safety, and research is continuing.

Be careful not to eat more of these products than what's recommended as safe. As set by the FDA, safety limits are sky high. It's almost inconceivable that the average person would exceed them. Take the current FDA maximum safe amount for aspartame, for example. It's 50 mg per kilogram of body weight per day. For a 132-lb. person, that translates to eighty packets of Equal or fifteen aspartame-sweetened soft drinks a day. That's a lot of aspartame! But if you consider that many other diet products contain aspartame, you could meet or exceed that limit in a day. So be careful. Canada is more conservative. The Canadian Diabetes Association sets its limit of aspartame at three to four packets of Equal or its equivalent a day.

Fake Fats

The fight against heart disease and the battle of the bulge have armed the food industry with newer nutritional weapons, namely fat replacers and fat substitutes. By mimicking fats and oils, these new products replace the real thing and trick your mouth into believing you're getting a high-fat treat, but without the calories.

Food technologists have discovered ways to concoct fake fats by changing the properties in everyday ingredients and making them feel and taste like fat in foods. Certain foods can be heated, acidified, and blended to resemble fat in all ways except two: They don't plug arteries, and they're low in calories.

Some fake fats—known as *fat replacers*—replace portions of fats in foods. Others take the place of fat altogether and are referred to as *fat substitutes*. Fat replacers and fat substitutes can be categorized as follows:

- Carbohydrate-based.
- Protein-based.
- Fat-based.

Carbo-hydrate-Based Fats

Used primarily as fat replacers, carbohydrate-based fats are formulated from starches and fibers. An example is polydextrose, a partially absorbable starch that supplies about 1 calorie per gram (versus 9 calories per gram from fat). Polydextrose is used in frozen desserts, puddings, and cake frostings. A similar product is maltodextrin, a starch made from corn. Containing 4 calories per gram, maltodextrin is used to replace fat in margarines and salad dressings.

Cellulose and gum are two types of fibers used to manufacture fat replacers. When ground into tiny particles, cellulose forms a consistency that feels like fat when eaten. Cellulose replaces some or all of the fat in certain dairy-type products, sauces, frozen desserts, and salad dressings. Gums such as xanthan gum, guar gum, pectin, and carageenan are used to thicken foods and give them a creamy texture. Added to salad dressings, desserts, and processed meats, gums cut the fat content considerably.

A newer carbohydrate-based fat replacer is Oatrim, developed by the U.S. Department of Agriculture for use in commercial baked foods and processed foods. Oatrim is made from the cholesterol-lowering soluble fiber in oat bran. In government studies, it lowered potentially dangerous levels of low-density lipoprotein (LDL) cholesterol by as much as 16 percent but without affecting levels of the beneficial high-density lipoprotein (HDL) cholesterol. Volunteers in the study also lost an average of 4.5 lb. during the ten-week research period.

Oatrim is used in Quaker Oats GatorBar and Healthy Choice hot dogs, ground beef, and cheeses. You can also find it sold as a powder for baking in some West Coast and Midwest supermarkets.

Protein-Based Fat Replacers

These are formulated from milk or eggs. One is the fat substitute Simplesse, made by Monsanto's NutraSweet division. Simplesse is created by heating and blending milk or egg white proteins into mistlike particles—technically known as microparticulated protein. Like real fat, these processed proteins feel creamy on the tongue. You digest and absorb Simplesse as if it were eggs and milk.

Depending on the formulation, Simplesse has 1 to 2 calories per gram. One drawback is that it can't be heated or it loses its desirable properties. However, it's ideal for frozen or refrigerated products. Simplesse is found in ice cream, yogurt, sour cream, dips, cheese spreads, salad dressings, mayonnaise, margarine, and butter spreads.

Other protein-based fat substitutes are Trailblazer, ULTRA-BAKE, ULTRA-FREEZE, and Lita, all concocted from milk, egg white, or corn proteins. These products are similar to microparticulated protein but are made from a different process. They're found in frozen desserts and baked goods.

Fat-Based Fat Replacers

When serving a fattening dessert, have you ever jokingly told your guests that "all the calories have been taken out"? It can be done! Food technologists have been hard at work trying to chemically change the properties of fats to remove or drastically cut fat calories. The result is fat-based fat replacers and fat substitutes. Some pass through the body unabsorbed, making them calorie-free. Others can even be used in cooking and frying, unlike carbohydrate- and protein-based fat replacers.

The carbohydrate- and protein-based fat replacers and substitutes just discussed all have FDA approval. But one of the fat-based fat replacers, Olestra (marketed as Olean) from Procter & Gamble, just received the government go-ahead with certain restrictions. Technically, Olestra is a *sucrose polyester,* meaning a combination of sugar and fatty acids. Your body can't digest Olestra, so it's classified as a noncaloric product.

According to the manufacturer, Olestra can be substituted for fats and oils in foods without loss of flavor. It has the same cooking properties as fats and oils and can be used in shortenings, oils, margarines, ice creams, desserts, and snacks. The original reports on the safety of Olestra indicated that it may block vitamin E absorption. Early formulations also caused diarrhea in some people, but improved versions have partially eliminated this problem, although some people

Table 20-1

KNOW YOUR ARTIFICIAL SWEETENERS AND FAKE FATS

Brand Name	Calories per Serving	Disadvantages
Artificial Sweetener		
Sweet'n Low/Sugar Twin (saccharin)	4	Bitter aftertaste; has been found to cause cancer in lab rats
Equal/NutraSweet (aspartame)	4	Destroyed during cooking; may cause reactions in people with sensitivity to the sweetener
Sunette (acesulfame-K)	0	Doesn't taste as much like sugar as the other sweeteners
Cyclamate	0	Lacks U.S. FDA approval; has been linked to cancer in lab rats
Artificial Fat		
Simplesse (processed proteins)	1–2 g	Can't be used for cooking
Oatrim (oat bran fiber)	1 g	Used in baked goods and processed foods
Olestra (sucrose polyester)	0	May cause diarrhea and loss of fat-soluable vitamins A, D, E, K, and B-carotene
Salatrim (processed vegetable oils)	3 g	Lacks FDA approval; still in development

may still get a laxative effect from its use. The FDA has restricted its use to snack foods. In addition, all Olestra products must be fortified with vitamins A, D, E, and K, and a required evaluation of the effect on the public will be conducted in 1998.

The latest entry into the fat-based fat replacer market is Salatrim from RJR Nabisco. Announced in 1994, this fake fat apparently tastes real but gives less than two-thirds the calories of conventional fat. Its makers say that once approved by the FDA, it can be used in everything from cheese to chocolate bars to cookies. Salatrim is formulated from vegetable oils and other foods.

The only fat-based fat replacers that have FDA approval to date are emulsifiers (which reduce fat and calories by replacing the shortening in cake mixes, cookies, icings, and other products) and caprenin (a cocoa butter–like ingredient used in candy). Caprenin has 5 calories per gram.

Recommendations for Using Sweeteners and Fake Fats

FDA approved or not, fat replacers and fat substitutes are being touted by the food industry as the final solution to winning the weight war. But I'm wary. Artificial sweeteners were launched by manufacturers using a similar strategy: By replacing the sugar in your diet with sweet substitutes, you could decrease your caloric intake and lose weight. But although many people try to cut calories by eating foods with artificial sugar, many others make up for it by eating twice as much. In fact, obesity is more prevalent in the United States than ever before.

Some fake fats are digested just like the unprocessed ingredients from which they come. Unless you're allergic to fake fats or their derivative foods, you shouldn't have any side effects. If you do have allergies, however, read the labels carefully to check for any "red flag" ingredients.

The key to enjoying any new fat-free product is to include it in your diet using a tried-and-true nutrition maxim—with moderation. Remember too, that even though a food may be fat-free, it's not necessarily calorie-free. Consult table 20-1 for information on the calorie counts and some of the disadvantages of the artificial fats and sweeteners. While indulging your tastes, don't forget to indulge your body's need for healthy ingredients, too.

CHAPTER 21

The Role of Exercise in Fat Loss

Exercise and Fat Burning

To lose body fat, you clearly have a lot of options. You can eat fewer calories and/or trim the fat from your diet. Or you can adjust your calories upward to spring yourself from starvation adaptation. But maybe you're unwilling to make dietary changes or cut back on your favorite foods. What's your best option now?

It's exercise specifically designed for maximum fat loss. I realize a lot of people reading this book are already very active and don't need to be told about the connection between exercise and weight control. But what you may not realize is that certain approaches to exercise are more effective than others for burning fat. You may need to make some changes in your exercise program—like doing more exercise, adding a strength-training component to your program, or gearing your aerobics to fat burning—to help you better control your weight. Let's look at how.

Burning Calories

The more exercise you do, the less you have to worry about calories. Remember, 1 lb. of body fat equals 3,500 calories. By burning 250 to 500 calories a day through exercise, you could lose up to a pound of fat a week (7 × 500 = 3,500)—without restricting food. If you need to lose extra body fat, either for health, appearance, or performance, the solution may be as simple as increasing your activity.

To help you in this regard, the energy cost of various activities is included in table 21-1. Each activity is described in terms of how many calories are burned each minute according to your weight. As an example, if you weigh 150 lb. and work out for forty-five minutes on a Nautilus strength-training program, you'd burn about 284 calories.

I'd like to emphasize that there's more to energy cost than just the calories burned during the activity. After you exercise, your metabolic rate stays elevated

Table 21-1

SELECTED EXAMPLES FOR ENERGY EXPENDITURES IN HOUSEHOLD, RECREATIONAL, AND SPORTS ACTIVITIES (IN CALORIES PER MINUTE)

Activity (calories per minute)	Your Body Weight In Pounds						
	117	**137**	**150**	**163**	**176**	**190**	**203**
Circuit training and free weights	4.5	5.8	5.6	6.3	6.8	7.4	7.8
Nautilus strength training	4.9	5.8	6.3	7.1	7.4	8.0	8.5
Cycling							
Leisure (5.5 mph)	3.4	4.0	4.4	4.7	5.1	5.5	5.9
Leisure (9.4 mph)	5.3	6.2	6.8	7.4	8.0	8.6	9.2
Dancing							
Aerobic, medium	5.5	6.4	7.0	7.6	8.2	8.9	9.5
Aerobic, intense	7.1	8.3	9.2	10.0	10.8	11.6	12.4
Gardening, mowing	5.9	6.9	7.6	8.3	9.0	9.6	10.3
Golf	4.5	5.3	5.8	6.3	6.8	7.3	7.8
Roller skating, leisure	6.2	7.3	8.0	8.6	9.3	10.1	10.8
Running (flat surface)							
11 min 30 sec/mile	7.2	8.4	9.2	10.0	10.9	11.7	12.6
9 min/mile	10.2	12.0	13.1	14.3	15.4	16.6	17.6
7 min/mile	12.7	14.5	15.6	16.8	17.9	19.1	20.8
Skiing, soft snow, leisure							
Women	5.2	6.1	6.7	7.3	7.8	8.4	9.0
Men	5.9	6.8	7.5	8.2	8.9	9.5	10.2
Swimming, crawl							
Fast	8.3	9.7	10.6	11.5	12.5	13.4	14.4
Slow	6.8	7.9	8.7	9.5	10.2	11.0	11.8
Tennis, recreational	5.8	6.8	7.4	8.1	8.7	9.4	10.0
Walking							
Leisure outdoors, asphalt road	4.2	5.0	5.4	5.9	6.4	6.9	7.4
Fields and hillsides	4.3	5.1	5.6	6.1	6.5	7.1	7.5
Treadmill (3.0 mph)	4.0	4.6	5.0	5.4	5.8	6.2	6.7

Used by permission. Copyright © by Frank I. Katch, Victor D. Katch, William McArdle, and Fitness Technologies, Inc., P.O. Box 430, Amherst, MA 01004. From F. I. Katch and W. D. McArdle, *Introduction to Nutrition, Exercise, and Health* (Malvern, PA: Lea & Febiger, 1993). No part of the tables may be reproduced in any form without written permission from the copyright holders.

for several hours, and you burn extra calories even at rest. And if you strength-train, you get even more of a metabolic boost: The muscle you develop is calorie-burning, metabolically active tissue. Having more of it cranks your metabolic rate up even higher.

Strength Training and Fat Loss

Perhaps your exercise of choice has always been aerobic activity, but you never seem to truly shape up. I know plenty of aerobic exercisers who have high percentages of body fat. Or maybe you're an endurance athlete who diets, only to lose valuable muscle and strength in the process.

No matter how active you are now or what your exercise of choice is, seriously consider starting a strength-training program. It may ultimately reprogram your resting metabolic rate so that your metabolism runs faster when you're not exercising. You're better able to burn off the calories you eat. What's more, strength training increases lean muscle tissue and decreases fat tissue. This alteration in body composition favors an elevation in your resting metabolic rate because muscle is metabolically more active than fat.

Strength training has a profound effect on metabolism, which is why I urge my non-strength-training clients to start. At Colorado State University, researchers recruited ten men, ages twenty-two to thirty-five, to see what effect, if any, strength training had on metabolism. At various times in the study, the men participated in strength training, aerobic exercise, or a control condition of quiet sitting. During the experiment, the subjects were fed controlled diets with a composition of 65 percent carbohydrate, 15 percent protein, and 20 percent fat.

In the strength-training portion of the experiment, the men performed a fairly standard yet strenuous routine: five sets of ten different upper and lower body exercises for a total of fifty sets. They worked out for about 100 minutes. As for aerobics, they cycled at moderate intensities for about an hour.

Exercise makes muscle cells hungry for oxygen. How much oxygen cells use is a chief indicator of whether metabolic rate has risen following exercise. In this study, the researchers measured oxygen usage with a technique called *indirect calorimetry*. This determines metabolic rate by analyzing oxygen uptake and carbon dioxide outflow, then calculating how much heat is produced. The more oxygen that's used following exercise, the higher the metabolic rate. Using this technique, RMR was measured the morning of exercise or sitting, and the morning following each experimental condition.

The findings: Strength training produced a higher rate of oxygen usage than either aerobics or quiet sitting, meaning that it was a better elevator of resting metabolic rate. In fact, the men's RMR stayed elevated for about fifteen hours after working out. Clearly, strength training won out as a metabolic booster and a calorie burner. If you strength-train, you'll have an easier time controlling your weight.

Lose Fat, Not Muscle, with Cross Training

A problem many weight-conscious exercisers and athletes have is losing too much muscle while dieting. If you lose 10 lb. of body weight, you may be lighter, but if five of those pounds are muscle, you sure won't be stronger, and your performance can really suffer. Appearance-wise, you can still look flabby when muscle tissue is lost. Cross training that includes strength training is one of the best ways to make sure you're shedding weight from fat stores rather than from lean muscle.

Researchers have put this principle to the test. In one study, 121 overweight women whose average age was fifty-three were placed in a diet-only group, a diet-plus-aerobic exercise and strength-training group, or a control group. The women in the diet-plus-exercise group worked out three times a week. Each workout included thirty minutes of aerobics (bicycling, stair stepping, or treadmill walking) and a strength-training period consisting of eight to ten exercises. The strength-training exercises worked all the major muscle groups.

After twelve weeks, it was time to check the results. Here's what happened: The diet-only group and the diet-plus-exercise group both lost weight, a loss that ranged from 6 to 40 lb. But more significantly, the composition of that loss was vastly different between groups. In the diet-plus-exercise group, women lost more fat—*and not a single ounce of lean muscle!*

What does all this tell us? Sure, you can lose weight by dieting alone. But you risk losing muscle. Not only that, your metabolic rate can plummet, sabotaging your attempts at successful weight control. By adding exercise (strength training and aerobics), you preserve calorie-burning muscle, hike your metabolism, and get in better shape, inside and out.

Two Ways to Maximize Your Aerobic Fat-Burning Potential

With aerobic exercise, there are two ways you can turn your body into a fat-burning machine: (1) intensity and (2) duration.

Intensity describes how hard you do your aerobics. At low-intensity exercise—twenty minutes or longer at around 50 percent of your maximum heart rate (220 minus your age*)—fat supplies as much as 90 percent of your fuel requirements.

Higher-intensity aerobics at roughly 75 percent of your maximum heart rate burns a smaller percentage of fat (around 60 percent) but results in more total calories burned overall, including more fat calories.

---

*For the average person, the MHR is 220, which refers to the maximum rate at which the heart can beat per minute. This decreases by one beat for every year of your life—unless you're a highly trained athlete. Elite athletes don't lose a beat. So if you're forty and not an elite athlete, your maximum heart rate is 180 (220 − 40 = 180). 50 percent of 180 is 90 beats a minute; 75 percent of 180 is 135 beats a minute.

To illustrate this concept, here's a comparison based on studies of aerobic intensity: At 50 percent, you burn 7 calories a minute, compared with 14 calories a minute at 75 percent. So at the 75 percent intensity, where 60 percent of the calories are from fat, you're burning 840 fat calories (60 × 14), compared with 630 fat calories (90 × 7). In short, you burn more total fat calories at higher intensities.

But unless you're in superb shape, it's difficult to exercise at a high intensity. You're better off exercising at a lower intensity for a longer period of time. That's what duration is all about: how long you exercise. You can burn just as much fat at a lower intensity by working out longer as you can exercising at a higher intensity for a shorter period of time.

To increase your rate of fat loss, gradually increase your aerobic exercise sessions from thirty to sixty minutes or striving for longer distances. For example, jogging a mile expends about 100 calories. Jog five miles, and you'll burn 500 calories. If you're jogging only a mile a day, it would take a month to lose a pound of fat, compared with about a week if you jog five miles a day.

Another option related to duration is frequency—working out more times a week to obtain a greater caloric expenditure. Perhaps you could add bicycling or swimming to your jogging program for some variety, along with the extra calorie burning. The real key is to enjoy whatever you do so that it becomes a lifelong habit.

Making Time to Exercise

Many exercisers and athletes are faced with lifestyle changes that interrupt their regular workout patterns. That's what happened to me after my daughter Danielle was born. Until then I had been a very active exerciser, with plenty of time for working out. With my daughter's birth, I realized my time wasn't my own anymore, especially with working and taking care of my family. It seemed I just didn't have time to work out. How could I preach the active lifestyle when I wasn't following it myself?

I set about to find ways to work exercise into my now-hectic schedule. In the winter, my husband and I started taking lots of long walks and hikes, with our baby bundled up papoose-style in a backpack I carried on my back. She just loved it. In the warmer months, I put her in a jogging stroller, and I'd walk or jog for long periods of time. My baby napped and I got my workout. Jogging strollers are great; they maneuver over harsh, bumpy terrain without a hitch.

As for my strength training, lifting a growing child is excellent progressive resistance exercise. My daughter weighed 7.5 lb. at birth, and three months later, she had doubled her weight to 15 lb. At a year old, she weighed 26 lb., and I was probably the strongest I'd ever been in terms of upper body strength, even though I had been strength training for years. Don't let anyone tell you that lifting barbells and dumbbells is the only way to build strength!

Table 21-2

STARTING A STRENGTH-TRAINING PROGRAM

- Consult your physician first and have a complete medical checkup before beginning any exercise program.
- Work under the guidance of a qualified personal trainer who can teach you proper technique and strength-training safety.
- Set realistic goals according to what you want to achieve: strength, muscular size, fat loss, prevention of bone loss, or a combination of these.
- Individualize your program, based on your goals.
- When designing a routine, include at least one exercise for each of your major body parts: thighs, chest, back, shoulders, arms, abdominals, and calves.
- Larger muscles—thighs, chest, and back—should be worked out early in your routine. This helps get your blood circulating faster. Plus, smaller muscles tire out faster. You need them to assist in larger-muscle exercises.
- When you first try an exercise, use a light weight—one that you can comfortably lift for about twelve repetitions. The last two to three repetitions should feel harder and require extra effort.
- On the lifting and lowering portion of an exercise, control the weight, without letting momentum take over.
- Perform two to three sets of each exercise. A set is a series of repetitions. Rest thirty seconds to one minute between exercise sets.
- Each time you exercise, work your way up. Strive to lift more weight than before or perform more repetitions. Progression builds strength and develops lean muscle.
- Breathe naturally as you exercise. Never hold your breath.
- Learn how to exercise using free weights (dumbbells and barbells) in addition to machine exercises. With free weights, more muscles are called into play. What's more, you can do literally hundreds of exercises with free weights, so you'll never get bored.
- Vary your workout by changing your choice of exercises, repetition, and intensity. Alter your routine if it's not producing the desired changes.
- Work out two to three times a week on nonconsecutive days. Your muscles need to rest approximately forty-eight hours before being exercised again.

I usually worked during Danielle's nap times. But several times a week, I'd use her nap time to pop in an exercise video and work out in front of the TV, keeping the volume low so as not to wake her up. There are lots of exercise videos on the market, and many are geared expressly for strength training. Some videos even teach you how to exercise with your baby. Before purchasing an exercise video,

Table 21-3

STARTING AN AEROBIC EXERCISE PROGRAM

- Consult your physician first and have a complete medical checkup before beginning any exercise program.

- Choose an aerobic activity that fits your present level of conditioning, lifestyle, and skill level.

- Begin your aerobic program gradually. Increase duration and intensity at regular intervals. The American College of Sports Medicine recommends exercising three or more times a week for twenty to sixty minutes each session. A twenty-minute session improves cardiovascular fitness. Aerobic activity that exceeds twenty minutes helps burn fat.

- Dress appropriately. Wear comfortable, loose-fitting clothing and proper shoes.

- Before and after exercise, take your heart rate—the number of times your heart beats for a full minute. Place the index and middle fingers of one hand about an inch away from your Adam's apple to find your carotid pulse. Then count the number of beats in a fifteen-second period and multiply by four.

- Stay within your target heart rate (THR) zone during exercise. To calculate this, find your maximum heart rate by subtracting your age from 220. Never exceed that number. Instead, try to stay within a range of 60 to 75 percent of that number. This is your target heart rate zone.

- Be sure to warm up and cool down properly.

- Stop exercising if you feel dizzy, faint, or short of breath.

check out the videos at your local library. Most libraries offer a good selection of exercise videos.

As my daughter has grown older—she'll be four soon—she loves to be outside, so we take walks. She rides her bicycle long distances, while I walk with her. Or I ride my bike and pull her behind me in her little trailer. I'm still lifting her periodically but not nearly as much as I had been. Now she's in a preschool program, which gives me more time to work out. Some days I run, other days I swim or lift weights. Because I still can't fit everything in, I try to combine aerobic exercise with strength training by running with handheld weights. This exercise combo has done wonders for my upper-body strength and cardiovascular fitness.

Even if you feel like you're not getting any exercise, you probably are, especially with housework, maintenance work around the home, gardening, or on-the-job labor. Before moving to Seattle, I used to live in a house where my laundry room and office were in the basement and the bedrooms on the second floor. I went up and down stairs all day. We moved to a home with no stairs, and after a few weeks, I really noticed a drop in my fitness level. The point is, you may be more active than you think, because of what you do around the house or at work.

Starting Your Program

If you're new to either strength training or aerobics, start slowly. For best results from exercise, the American College of Sports Medicine recommends engaging in aerobic exercise for twenty to sixty minutes three or more times a week, along with strength training two to three times a week. To increase your strength, you must challenge your muscles to work harder each time you exercise. That means a gradual increase in poundages from workout to workout. With aerobics, increase your intensity gradually, too. Your goal should be to work out hard enough aerobically to burn as much fat as you can.

Before you begin any exercise program, consult your physician. Once you begin, be sure to work with someone well trained and familiar with both aerobic and strength-training programs. Tables 21-2 and 21-3 provide important guidelines for starting a strength-training and aerobics program.

CHAPTER 22

If You Want to Maintain or Gain Weight

Overcoming Yo-Yo Dieting

Dieters often fall into the trap of the dieting-rebound cycle, also known as yo-yo dieting, in which weight is lost and regained continually. Going on and off diets like this can make you fatter than ever. As weight is continually lost, especially with unsafe practices such as drastic calorie cutting, more lean muscle is lost. When you regain weight after dieting, a lot of it is fat tissue. These shifts dramatically alter your body composition in favor of fat and lower your resting metabolic rate. The key is to become a maintainer, not a regainer, after you've reached your healthy body weight.

Becoming a Maintainer

How do you do that? Success or failure at losing weight depends on several factors: fat intake, diet, exercise patterns, and social support. Here's why I say that: A group of dietitians decided to explore just what makes people take off weight, then keep it off. They collected data from people who had participated in a work-site weight control program held at a Midwestern university campus between 1987 and 1990. Six months long, this particular program was behaviorally oriented. The dieters met once a week for an hour for the first six to eight weeks, and then twice a month for the remaining six months. Fourteen men and fifteen women participated in the study.

Information from the dieters was taken both six months and forty-two months after completing the program. The dieters filled out questionnaires that asked them about their diet; weight loss and regain patterns; exercise habits; and social support from spouse, children, friends, and coworkers. Measurements such as weight and height were taken as well.

Some interesting findings emerged from both follow-ups:

- Twenty of the dieters had regained weight. Of significance was that these regainers had a chronic history of yo-yo dieting.

- Eleven of the regainers and four of the maintainers were women.
- Regainers (both men and women) ate more of their calories at dinner than the maintainers did.
- The nine dieters who had maintained their weight tended to eat less total fat. Plus, they exercised more and for longer periods of time.
- There was no strong correlation between social support and the ability to maintain a healthy weight—probably a result of the small sample size. The researchers emphasized that social support is still an important factor in weight control.

Tips for Keeping Weight Off

In working with people who have dieted and then kept their weight off, I've developed several important tips that will help you do the same:

- Keep your fat intake in the 20 to 25 percent range of total daily calories.
- Consider eating your heaviest meals earlier in the day. Big evening meals tend to be metabolized when you're sleeping, a time when calories can turn into fat more easily. Eat higher-calorie meals earlier in the day. There's a better chance they'll be burned off by exercise and other activities.
- If you have a history of yo-yo dieting, put your weight loss desires aside for a while. Focus instead on becoming more active and reducing fat in your diet by increasing carbohydrates. Both measures will help you become more fit with the least amount of trouble.
- Social support helps. Enlist the help of your family, friends, and co-workers in making lifestyle changes.
- Exercise, exercise, exercise. Enough said!

Gaining Weight

In a society obsessed with losing weight, you've probably been lost in the shuffle if you want to gain weight. Without any good information on gaining weight, maybe you've devised your own strategy. For some of you, that might have meant loading up on ice cream, milkshakes, and other goodies. The problem is, weight gain diets like that add too much fat. And that opens the door to obesity, clogged arteries, heart disease, cancer, and other life-shortening illnesses.

Is there a healthy way to gain weight? You bet, and it involves a high-carbohydrate diet combined with strength training. This combination helps you build lean, toned, tight muscle, rather than flabby fat.

To gain quality weight (and that means muscle), you need to eat more calories than your body needs to maintain its weight. But you must choose those calories wisely. In chapter 5, we saw how protein plays a role in gaining lean muscle. But protein is only part of the story.

Carbohydrates figure in, too, and research bears this out. In Denver, researchers looked into the effects of a liquid high-calorie diet supplement on diet, weight gain, body composition, and strength on a group of nine competitive weight lifters. A group of ten control weight lifters were studied in the same manner but were not given the supplement. All the subjects ate their regular diets to maintain their weight gain goals.

Those subjects taking the supplement gained significantly more weight than the controls: 3.5 lb. more. In fact, the supplement group gained twice the lean body mass compared with the controls. Interestingly, the supplement group lost .9 percent body fat. Strength gains were greater in the supplement group compared with the controls.

When their diets were analyzed, subjects in the supplement group ate about 830 calories more a day than the controls. Subjects in the control group ate more of their calories from fat (45 percent fat and 37 percent carbs) than the supplement group, whose diet was 34 percent fat and 47 percent carbs. Even if you don't consider yourself a weight lifter, this research still makes it clear that you can build muscle safely by eating plenty of calories, especially when most of them are carb calories.

Building a Pound of Muscle

It takes energy to do the exercise that builds muscle. You need to eat at least the amount of calories you burn to keep your weight as it is—and more calories to gain. To build a pound of muscle, add on 2,500 extra calories a week. That means introducing 400 to 500 calories a day (or 12 to 25 calories per pound of body weight a day) to compensate for your extra exercise. But don't get carried away and eat too much too soon. Gradually increase your calories for a slow but steady gain. Trying to gain too fast leads to unhealthy, unsightly body fat.

Remember: 65 to 70 percent of your calories should come from carbohydrates. Carbs fuel your muscles for exercise and help promote muscular development. What's more, carb calories increase the chance that your weight gain is pure muscle, not fat. Be sure to refuel your muscles with some carbs immediately after exercise to recharge yourself for future workouts. Also, eat or drink additional high-carbohydrate foods within thirty minutes to two hours after each workout. As for protein, eat .7 g of protein per pound of body weight a day. On a high-carb diet, your protein intake will make up only 10 to 12 percent of your total calories for the day. The rest of your diet, 25 percent or less of your calories, comes from fat. You won't have to worry too much about your fat intake as long as you concentrate on eating enough carbohydrates to meet your energy needs.

Getting Enough Calories

Between working, sleeping, and exercising, you might have trouble eating all the calories required on a weight-gaining diet. Here are a couple of strategies to help you:

✔ *Even if you have to eat them on the run, be sure to eat all your meals.* Skipping even one meal a day will throw your weight gain plan off course. On-the-run breakfast options include a bagel spread with peanut butter and jelly or toasted cheese on an English muffin. You can nibble on these while sitting in your car at a traffic light or on your way to the bus stop. If you commute by train, you might try packing a full breakfast of cereal, fruit, and yogurt to eat during your ride. Yogurt works great in place of spilly milk.

✔ *Give in to snack attacks.* Snacking is a critical part of gaining weight. You can sneak in extra calories you've missed at meals. Snacks are like little meals, and you may need three or more a day to meet your goals. One of the easiest snacks is a meal replacement sports drink. But don't use meal replacers for more than one meal or one snack a day. They don't have all the components of food and should never be used to replace food on a regular basis.

Go Slowly to Achieve Healthy Body Composition Changes

Don't get discouraged by slow changes on the scale or in your circumference measurements. The slower your weight loss or gain, the better. A slow loss indicates you're losing weight from fat stores; a slow gain means you're putting on lean muscle, not fat. Both changes indicate that your shape, as well as your health, is changing for the better.

PART SEVEN

NUTRITION FOR SPECIAL NEEDS

CHAPTER 23

High-Performance Vegetarian Nutrition

The Popularity of Vegetarian Diets

If you're like me, you probably grew up with meat as the centerpiece of your meals. Now we know that eating too much meat and other animal flesh has some proven health risks. By contrast, a meatless diet may serve up a menu for long life by preventing many chronic diseases, from cancer to heart disease. If you exercise regularly or play sports, a vegetarian diet can give you the extra pep you need to perform, plus supply the vital nutrients you need to develop lean muscle tissue.

At present, vegetarians make up about 7 percent of the population or about 12.4 million people. I expect this number to grow as more Americans discover that a meat-centered diet may not be the healthiest.

Types of Vegetarians

The term *vegetarian* refers to people with a range of eating habits:

- *Semi-vegetarians* eat dairy foods, eggs, poultry, and fish but avoid red meat.
- *Pesco-vegetarians* eat dairy foods, eggs, and fish but no other animal flesh.
- *Lacto-ovo-vegetarians* eat dairy foods and eggs but exclude animal flesh from their diets.
- *Lacto-vegetarians* eat dairy foods but no eggs or animal flesh.
- *Ovo-vegetarians* eat eggs but no dairy foods or animal flesh.
- *Total vegetarians,* or *vegans,* eat no animal foods of any type.

B Vitamins in Vegetarian Meals

Clearly, vegetarian diets vary widely. If you're thinking of becoming a vegetarian, the trick is to make sure you're not skimping on any nutrients when you cut out certain foods (see table 23-2). Vegans run the greatest risk of deficiencies because several vital nutrients are found only in meat, eggs, and dairy products. Vitamin B_{12} is one. Fortunately, the body needs very tiny amounts of B_{12} daily to do its job of helping manufacture red blood cells and nerves.

Even so, a deficiency is serious, potentially causing irreversible nerve damage. Numbness or tingling in the arms or legs, memory loss, weakness, and incoordination are the first signs of nerve impairment from a vitamin B_{12} deficiency. The body's B_{12} stores can be depleted by prolonged stress, use of birth control pills, heavy menstrual periods, and any illness that damages the intestinal lining, where this vitamin is absorbed. Plus, the need for vitamin B_{12} increases during pregnancy and breast feeding.

Eating fermented foods, such as the soybean products miso and tempeh, supplies some vitamin B_{12} from the bacterial culture that causes fermentation but generally not enough. I advise vegans to eat vitamin B_{12}-fortified foods or take supplements to ensure a healthy diet. The supplement should contain 100 percent of the RDA or 2 μg of vitamin B_{12}.

Vegetarian diets are often short on riboflavin, a B vitamin involved in the metabolism of carbohydrates, fats, and proteins. Brewer's yeast, green leafy vegetables, and enriched breads and cereals are good sources of riboflavin. Adding dairy products to the diet supplies riboflavin, too.

Mining for More Minerals

Most vegetarians get enough minerals in their diets—with the exception of calcium, iron, and zinc. These minerals are often in short supply in many vegetarian diets, since they're found abundantly in meats and dairy products. Here's how to make sure you get enough of essential minerals in a vegetarian diet.

Calcium   The RDA for calcium is 800 mg for men, 1,200 mg for women, and 1,500 mg for postmenopausal women. Unfortunately, the body has a hard time absorbing calcium. One factor that helps is drinking milk. As noted in chapter 8, milk contains a sugar called lactose, which stimulates the absorption of calcium from the intestine. By getting your calcium from milk rather than from supplements, you get more calcium per swallow. In fact, milk-drinking vegetarians probably don't need to supplement. Research shows that they get enough calcium and rarely have bone density problems.

Some people are sensitive to lactose—a condition called lactose intolerance — and can't drink milk without getting an upset stomach. Studies show that people who are lactose intolerant tend to have less calcium in their diets and less bone mass. No one knows yet whether this reduction in bone density is due to a low-calcium diet or some other complication of the lactose intolerance. But it's clear that more calcium in the diet would be helpful. If you have problems digesting milk, try using the lactase enzyme replacers, such as Lactaid and Dairyease. These should help you add more milk to your diet. Or include yogurt in your diet, which might be more easily digested if you're lactose intolerant. Check the label to make sure it contains live active yogurt cultures (*L. bulgaricus, S. thermophilus,* or *L. acidophilus*). These will digest some of the lactose, can destroy dangerous food-borne bacteria, and have protective effects against disease.

Not all vegetarians drink milk or eat yogurt, however, and are therefore at risk of a calcium deficiency. To prevent a shortfall, vegans and ovo-vegetarians should include alternative sources of this bone-building mineral in their diets such as broccoli, collard greens, kale, dark leafy vegetables, tofu, fortified soy milk, and calcium-fortified fruit juice (see table 23-1). Often it's difficult to get enough calcium from these sources, so a calcium supplement should be taken each day.

Where a calcium deficiency exists, there may also be a vitamin D shortage. Milk is routinely fortified with vitamin D, which assists in the absorption of calcium in the intestines. If you drink milk, you're automatically getting a vitamin D supplement. Sunlight activates a substance in the skin and turns it into vitamin D, so most people get enough from regular exposure to the sun. For vegetarians who don't eat dairy products and have limited time in the sun, a supplement providing 100 percent of the RDA or 5 µg of vitamin D is good insurance.

Iron

Nutritionally, there are two types of iron: *heme* iron, found only in beef, poultry, and fish; and *nonheme* iron, found mostly in vegetables and grains. The body doesn't absorb nonheme iron as well as it absorbs iron from animal foods. Only about 5 percent of the nonheme iron is taken up by the body compared with 25 percent for heme iron. Even though vegetarians may be eating enough iron from plants and grains, they may not be absorbing enough of it for good health.

Fortunately, the absorption of nonheme iron is enhanced by what's eaten with it. Vitamin C–rich foods such as oranges, orange juice, grapefruits, and other fruits can more than double the amount of iron absorbed. In fact, vegetarians should eat foods containing vitamin C at every meal. Those who think their diets may be iron-deficient should consider supplementing with a one-a-day type mineral supplement containing 100 percent of the RDA (10 mg of iron for men and 15 mg for women).

Zinc

Zinc is plentiful in seafood but is also present in whole grains, peas, corn, and carrots. Vegetarians often have low levels of zinc, and one explanation is their high

Table 23-1

ALTERNATE SOURCES OF CALCIUM FOR MILK-FREE DIETS

Amount	Food	Mg of Calcium
½ cup	Collard greens, cooked	152
1 cup	Soy milk (fortified)	150
2 oz.	Mackerel, canned	148
½ cup	Dandelion greens, cooked	140
½ cup	Turnip greens, cooked	139
½ cup	Mustard greens, cooked	138
½ cup	Kale, cooked	125
2–6″	Tortillas	120
1 tbsp.	Blackstrap molasses	116
1 large	Orange	96
2 oz.	Salmon, canned	88
2 medium	Sardines, canned	88
½ cup	Boston baked beans	85
2 oz.	Herring, canned	84
½ cup	Soybeans, cooked	73
½ cup	Broccoli	66
½ cup	Rutabagas, cooked	59
1	Artichoke, cooked	51
½ cup	White beans, cooked	50
½ cup	Kidney beans, cooked	48
12–15 nuts	Almonds	38
1 oz.	Tofu	36

Source: Heath, M. K. ed. 1982. *Diet Manual. Including a Vegetarian Meal Plan,* 6th ed. Seventh-Day Adventist Dietetic Association, P.O. Box 75, Loma Linda, CA 92345.

intake of *phytates.* Phytates are natural substances found in certain vegetables, including whole grains, beet greens, lentils, and eggplant. They block the absorption of both zinc and iron. If you eat a lot of foods high in phytates, supplementing with zinc might be a good idea. Take a mineral supplement that has 100 percent of the RDA for zinc (15 mg for men and 12 mg for women).

Vegetarian Protein

As discussed in chapter 5, animal proteins contain the nine essential amino acids needed for good health. Your body can't make these. You have to get them from your diet. When a food contains all the essential amino acids, it's called a complete protein. Animal foods are complete protein sources. Plant foods, on the other hand, are termed incomplete protein sources because they may be high in some of the essential amino acids but low in others.

To get enough essential amino acids from a vegetarian diet, you have to mix and match foods during the day so that those low in an essential amino acid are balanced by one that's higher in the same amino acid (see table 23-2). Certain cultures have developed traditional dishes that often combine several foods that complement each other to create complete proteins. Combining beans with grains or flour, such as beans and rice, corn tortillas and refried beans, or pasta and bean soup, creates a fully nutritious protein meal.

Lacto-ovo-vegetarians, however, needn't worry about piecing together complete proteins from foods. The protein in the eggs, milk, and dairy products they eat has all the essential amino acids. The only catch is dietary fat. Some dairy products are too high in artery-clogging fat. Protein-rich plant sources, low-fat and nonfat milk, cheeses, and yogurts should be the protein fare of choice. Egg

Table 23-2

HOW TO MEET NUTRIENT NEEDS THE VEGETARIAN WAY

Nutrient	Sources
Protein	Legumes combined with grains or seeds; any plant food combined with eggs or dairy products
Calcium	Dairy products, dark leafy greens, fortified soy milk, legumes, peanuts, almonds, seeds, and calcium-fortified fruit juice
Iron	Legumes, dark leafy vegetables, torula yeast, dried fruits, whole and enriched grains, cooking in cast iron pots. Consuming foods that contain vitamin C (citrus fruits, peppers, tomatoes) with any iron-rich food will improve absorption.
Zinc	Whole-grain products, brewer's yeast, wheat bran, wheat germ, and pumpkin seeds
Vitamin B_{12}	Dairy products, eggs, nutritional yeast, foods fortified with B_{12}, fermented soy products, and supplements
Riboflavin	Dairy products, eggs, whole and enriched grains (if eaten in large quantities) brewer's yeast, dark green leafy greens, and legumes
Vitamin D	Fortified milk, fortified soy milk, and exposure of the skin to sunshine

yolks should be limited to three to four a week. Virtually all the protein in eggs is found in the whites, anyway.

Beans—A Healthy Staple of Vegetarian Diets

Remember this ditty? "Beans, beans, the musical fruit. The more you eat, the more you toot."

Today kids sing: "Beans, beans, they're good for your heart / The more you eat, the more you . . ."

How times have changed. Now even kids know that beans—a vegetarian mainstay—are a healthy food. But if you're like a lot of people, you tend to shy away from them because of their gas-producing side effects. New discoveries on the health power of beans, however, are overshadowing their drawbacks.

Technically, dry beans are categorized as legumes and include beans, peas, and lentils. There are thirteen thousand kinds of legumes, but humans use only about twenty as food. Among those twenty, there's a wide variety of colors, sizes, shapes, and flavors. Calorie-wise though, most dry beans are similar. A half-cup serving provides between 110 and 143 calories of energy-giving carbohydrates.

Some legumes, such as soybeans and peanuts, are cultivated for both their protein and their oil content. Others, like lentils, lima beans, chickpeas, and peas, are grown for their value as protein sources. In either case, dry beans are among the most nourishing of all vegetables.

Beans are also loaded with water-soluble vitamins, especially thiamin, riboflavin, niacin, and folic acid. Canned beans, however, may be lower than home-cooked beans due to processing. Beans are also mineral-rich, full of calcium, iron, copper, zinc, phosphorus, potassium, and magnesium. But there's a hitch: Minerals in beans aren't absorbed as well as minerals from animal foods. Nonetheless, the other amazing health benefits of beans truly outweigh this minor shortcoming.

If you're trying to cut down on fat while keeping a healthy amount of protein in your diet, beans are for you. The fat content of beans is very low, ranging from 0.8 to 1.5 percent. The two exceptions are soybeans (19 percent) and peanuts (46 percent). The fat is mostly from unsaturated fat, and there's not a smidgen of cholesterol in beans.

On average, 21 to 25 percent of the calories in beans come from protein. Soybeans are the exception, with about 34 percent of their calories coming from protein. Another plus: You'll pay less for the protein in beans than you will for any other source of protein.

The protein quality in beans, however, does have some limitations. Compared with animal foods, the proteins in beans are not as completely digested. Even so, well-processed soybean protein equals the protein quality in animal foods.

Few foods are as rich in carbs as beans. The total carbohydrate content of most dried beans ranges from about 60 to 65 g in each half-cup serving and is mostly starch. Other carbs include fiber. The total fiber of cooked dry beans is 4 to 7 g in a serving.

The fiber of note in beans is the water-soluble type, known to lower blood cholesterol and keep blood glucose in safe bounds. Just a half a cup to a full cup of beans daily can significantly cut cholesterol and control blood sugar. Beans also contain a significant amount of insoluble fibers. These aid in proper elimination and are linked to a decreased risk of colon cancer.

A small amount of the carbs in beans comes from sugars, namely raffinose, stachyose, and verabose. These sugars are the culprits in the intestinal problems associated with beans. The small intestine doesn't have the right enzymes to digest these sugars, so they arrive in the large intestine undigested. Bacteria residing there have a heyday feeding off these sugars and fermenting them. Carbon dioxide, hydrogen, and other gases are given off in the process.

Eliminating Gas from Beans

You can put a stop to most of the gas-producing problem by following a few easy steps:

- Soak the beans for four to five hours (overnight or during the day while you're at work), and discard the soaking water afterward.
- Add fresh water. For best results, add 9 cups of water for every cup of beans. Bring the water to a boil for ten minutes, and then simmer for thirty minutes. Again, toss out the water.
- If the beans still require cooking, add more water and simmer. Discard this water as well. Most beans require approximately one to two hours of cooking.

You can relieve any remaining discomfort caused by undigested sugars by using a product called Beano (AkPharma Inc.), an enzyme preparation that does the digesting for you. Beano will also help reduce intestinal gas caused by high-fiber vegetables like cabbage, broccoli, and brussels sprouts.

If You're a Physically Active Vegetarian

On average, vegetarians who eat no flesh foods take in fewer calories than meat eaters, semi-vegetarians, or pesco-vegetarians. The reason is, their diets contain less total fat and protein. The vegetarian diet is typically very nutrient-rich, however, because of the quality of foods eaten. Vegetarians who are very active should make sure they're eating enough calories to fuel their energy needs. One solution is to choose higher-calorie foods such as beans, potatoes, yams, pasta, dried fruits, nuts, and seeds.

To get enough calories and nutrients, vegetarians should eat between 1,800 and 3,000 calories a day, with the minimum number of servings (appendix A contains information on what constitutes a serving size) from the following food groups:

Semi-vegetarians, pesco-vegetarians, and lacto-ovo-vegetarians:
- 6–11 servings of bread, cereal, rice, and pasta
- 3–5 servings of vegetables
- 2–4 servings of fruit
- 2–3 servings of milk, yogurt, and cheese
- 2–3 servings of poultry, fish, dried beans, eggs, and nuts

Lacto-vegetarians:
- 8–11 servings of bread, cereal, rice, and pasta
- 3–5 servings of vegetables
- 3–4 servings of fruit
- 2–3 servings of milk and yogurt
- 1–2 servings of low-fat cheese
- 4–6 servings of dried beans and peas
- 2–4 servings of nuts and seeds

Vegans:
- 8–11 servings of bread, cereal, rice, and pasta
- 4–6 servings of vegetables
- 3–4 servings of fruit
- 6–8 servings of dried beans and peas
- 3–5 servings of nuts and seeds

Vegetarians and Physical Performance

Let's say you make the switch to a vegetarian diet. Will your exercise performance suffer? What about your energy levels? Can you still develop body-firming muscle, even though you're not eating animal protein?

Put your fears aside. Vegetarian diets are typically high in carbohydrates and low in fat. That's perfect for exercisers and athletes. With 60 percent to 70 percent of your diet coming from carb-packed grains, beans, fruits, and vegetables, there's no way your performance will drop off.

Studies have confirmed this, and that's why I wholeheartedly support vegetarian diets for all active people. For example, during a six-week experimental period, investigators compared the endurance output of two sets of endurance athletes: those on a mixed meat-rich diet and those who switched to a lacto-ovo-vegetarian diet. The changeover to a vegetarian diet didn't harm performance at all.

Strength trainers often worry whether they can still develop muscle on a meatless diet. The good news is that you can can definitely develop lean muscle as a vegetarian. Here's some proof: In one study, people who ate a high-carbohydrate, moderate-protein diet during training gained significantly more muscle than their counterparts who ate high-protein diets.

Many world-class athletes are vegetarians who credit their success to nutrition. One is Bill Pearl, a four-time Mr. Universe who became a vegetarian (lacto-ovo) nearly thirty years ago after finding out that his cholesterol had dangerously surpassed the 300 mark. He went on to win two of his Mr. Universe titles as a vegetarian while scaling his cholesterol down to 200. Pearl is still a vegetarian today.

I once worked with an NBA basketball player who for philosophical reasons decided to become a lacto-vegetarian. Very determined, he wanted to know how he could stick to his vegetarian game plan, both on the road and at home.

Unexpectedly, this player's biggest problem was not protein. He was getting plenty of protein from eating dairy products. But he wasn't getting enough iron, selenium, and zinc—minerals that are plentiful in flesh foods. Also, his diet was very high in fat, since he was eating a lot of cheese-laden vegetable lasagna.

To solve the mineral problem, I recommended that he take a mineral supplement containing the RDAs of the minerals he was lacking. After basketball practice, he began drinking one or two meal replacement beverages. These contain extra nutrients and can be used by lacto-vegetarians.

We found lots of low-fat recipes, like vegetarian chili, that could be packed for road trips and eaten for dinner, as long as he had a microwave oven in his hotel room. He took dried fruit along, too. An eat-anywhere snack, dried fruit is loaded with nutrients and energy-packed calories.

He needed to round out his diet at home for more variety. I planned his nutrition program using vegetarian staples such as beans, tofu, rice, and peanut butter. He started eating a lot of different foods while still getting plenty of quality calories to fuel his very active lifestyle. Equally important, he learned he could be a strict lacto-vegetarian, in keeping with his beliefs, and do it successfully.

Benefits of a Vegetarian Lifestyle

For the prevention-minded, the ultimate payoff of a vegetarian lifestyle is long-term health. Vegetarians live longer, healthier lives, with less disease. The evidence in support of this is convincingly strong, as discussed in the next sections.

Kill Off Obesity

Obesity plays dangerous games with your body. It increases your chance of heart disease by 50 percent, more than doubles a man's risk of getting prostate cancer, and ups the risk of colon cancer three times. Not a pleasant picture, no matter how you look at it.

Part of the problem is the high fat content in animal foods. Your body stores dietary fat much more readily than it does carbohydrate. The more fat you eat, the more you're likely to wear. On average, vegetarian diets tend to be low in fat, so it stands to reason that vegetarians are trimmer. Take the Chinese, for example. Researchers are convinced the Chinese are lean because they eat two-thirds less fat than Americans and double the starchy foods.

Then there's the fiber factor. Vegetarian diets are loaded with fiber, which helps you lose weight and keep it off. Exactly how fiber does this is unclear, although there are some theories. One is that fiber "dilutes" calories by shortening the time it takes for food to move through the intestines, and this decreases its absorption. Another is that fiber takes longer to digest in the stomach. You feel full as a result, with fewer hunger pangs. One interesting study found that eating a high-fiber cereal at breakfast makes you eat less at lunch, cutting your daily calorie intake. Given its many benefits, a vegetarian diet is an excellent way to control body weight, prevent obesity, and dodge its potentially fatal health problems.

Unplug Arterial Pipes

The higher your cholesterol, the greater your chance of plaque buildup inside your artery walls. You can help circumvent this problem with a low-fat, fiber-rich diet. As mentioned, vegetarian diets are low in saturated fat and high in fiber—two factors that lower dangerous LDL cholesterol. Vegetarians eat two to three times more fiber than nonvegetarians—and are healthier for it. Eating more soluble fiber from oats, dried beans, and legumes keeps harmful cholesterol at bay.

Stay Heart Healthy

Many studies have proved that a low-fat vegetarian diet not only prevents heart disease, it also can reverse it. In one study, a low-fat, near-vegan diet combined with daily exercise and a stress management program, had dramatic effects on the heart health of patients. After a year, eighteen of the twenty-two patients in the study showed significant clearing in their arteries, plus a 91 percent reduction in the frequency of chest pains.

Nonvegetarian men in their forties are four times more likely to have heart attacks than vegetarians. Overall, vegetarians have a much lower risk of heart attacks, strokes, and other circulatory diseases. The reason has to do with saturated fat and cholesterol, which are so much lower in vegetarian diets than in meat-based diets.

Fight Cancer

The connection between cancer and diet is becoming stronger all the time. In fact, the medically accepted guidelines for reducing cancer risk sound like a dietary road map for vegetarians. For example:

- Reduce your fat consumption to no more than 30 percent of your total calories.
- Increase the amount of fiber and whole grain cereals in your diet.
- Eat more fruits and vegetables (besides fiber, these are loaded with vitamin A, beta-carotene, and vitamin C, all known to have a cancer-protective effect).
- Eat fewer cured and smoked meats (these contain nitrites and fat, both linked to cancer risk).
- Limit your consumption of charcoal-broiled foods (outdoor cooking can release cancer-causing substances).

The cancer-fighting benefits of a vegetarian-type diet (low-fat/high-fiber) are clearest in cancers of the colon and rectum. Many studies show a strong association between high-meat diets and colon cancer. Experts theorize that bile and fatty acids, by-products of the meat-digestion process, play a part in tumor growth. In one study, subjects who changed from a meat diet to a lacto-vegetarian diet had 75 percent less bile and fatty acids following a three-month period of vegetarian eating than those who ate meat.

Other research has turned up these findings: Meat eaters have a 28 percent higher risk of breast cancer, a 51 percent higher risk of prostate cancer, and a 66 percent higher risk of ovarian cancer. A study of Japanese men found that those who ate meat every day had 2.5 times the rate of pancreatic cancer than those who were vegetarians.

Diet against Diabetes

A high-carbohydrate, low-fat diet is the standard dietary prescription for diabetes—and for good reason. This type of diet helps fight obesity, which is associated with Type II diabetes. Plus, its high-fiber content helps regulate glucose. As well, eating a carb-rich diet helps make the body more sensitive to insulin.

A case in point is the Pima Indians of southern Arizona. For centuries the Pimas ate traditional native foods: prickly pears, beans, wolfberries, mustard seeds, and other wild and cultivated plants. In the late 1930s their diet began to change. Members of the tribe migrated outside the reservation for jobs and began to taste modern foods. Pima men served in World War II and ate K rations. Peanut butter, cheeses, butter, and meat were donated to the reservation by the government. Gradually, hamburgers, white bread, and other high-fat, sugary foods replaced the native diet.

Today more than half the Pimas over age thirty-five have Type II diabetes. Researchers probed this epidemic and learned that the Pimas are genetically vulnerable to developing this type of diabetes. Evidently, eating sugary, high-fat, overprocessed foods triggered the disease.

The Pimas' native foods were analyzed by a nutritionist and tested on healthy nondiabetics. What followed is eye-opening: The traditional native foods slowed carbohydrate digestion and dramatically lowered insulin production and glucose levels. These foods prevented the dangerous bodily responses people with Type II diabetes need to steer clear of: sharp rises in insulin and blood sugar.

Out with Osteo-porosis

Diets high in animal protein can cause calcium to leach out of the bones and not be reabsorbed, says a University of Texas study. The researchers added eggs and meat to the diets of vegans and observed that their risk of developing osteoporosis went up. Another study looked at a group of Eskimos who eat up to 400 g of protein a day (primarily from fish). Even though they get as much as 2,500 mg of calcium a day, their rate of bone loss and osteoporosis was much greater than that of Caucasian Americans. More proof that bones can stay protected with a vegetarian diet: Osteoporosis is rare in China, where the Chinese get most of their calcium from vegetables.

Live Longer   Vegetarians live longer than people who eat meat-containing diets. That's one conclusion of a thirty-year study of fifty thousand Seventh-Day Adventists. By religious belief, Seventh-Day Adventists exclude meat, fish, and eggs from their diets. Compared with the general population, Adventist men live 8.9 years longer; Adventist women, 7.5 years longer.

The longer you're a vegetarian, the better off you are, according to a study of 1,900 German vegetarians. Those who were vegetarians for twenty or more years had a lower risk of death—a great testimony to the protective nature of this lifestyle.

Making the Switch to Vegetarianism

Suppose you decide to give vegetarianism a shot. What changes could you reasonably expect in a year's time? Based on what we know, here are some possibilities

Your cholesterol profile would change favorably, perhaps within a week. When volunteers went on an uncooked, "living food" vegetarian diet for seven days, their cholesterol levels dropped significantly. Also, concentrations of vitamin E and vitamin A increased in their blood.

If you drink more milk for protein, you'll boost your intake of bone-building calcium. Your elimination would be better, since you'd be eating more fiber. Plus, you'd have more energy because of the carbohydrate volume in your diet. And as long as you stick to low-fat and nonfat dairy products, you should shed any excess body fat. There's no question that many positive changes would take place very early on.

How should you make the switch? Excuse the pun, but it's best not to go "cold turkey" when quitting your meat-based diet. Most people find it easier to phase into vegetarian eating by becoming a partial vegetarian. Do this with a gradual reduction in the amount of meat you eat. For example, plan several meatless days each week or a meatless meal each day. Another strategy is to become a semi-vegetarian or a pesco-vegetarian before moving on to the stricter forms of vegetarianism.

To help you make the switch, here are some additional pointers:

- For starters, eliminate red meat, but continue to eat poultry and fish occasionally.
- Make complex carbohydrates rather than an animal protein the centerpiece of your meals.
- Early on, incorporate one vegetarian meal a day into your menus, eventually phasing out flesh foods and making all meals vegetarian.
- Because vegetarian diets are high in fiber, they add bulk to the diet. Too much too soon, however, leads to intestinal discomfort. Gradually introduce high-fiber foods into your diet.

- Find vegetarian recipes you enjoy.
- Consider "substitute meats"—products made from soybeans that are formed to look and taste like hot dogs, sausage, ground beef, and bacon.
- For variety and good health, include many different foods, since no single food contains all the nutrients you need.

If changing to a vegetarian style of eating, you may want to seek out a registered dietitian to make sure your diet is healthy and well balanced. This is especially critical during pregnancy, breast feeding, or recovery from an illness. Call your local dietetic association or hospital for referrals. Another excellent resource is the National Center for Nutrition and Dietetics Consumer Nutrition Hotline at (800) 366-1655.

CHAPTER 24

Nutrition during Pregnancy

Prepregnancy Nutrition

I'm always excited when a client of mine says she would like to start eating right before she gets pregnant rather than waiting until she's already pregnant. Your nutritional health is cumulative: How well your body feeds your baby and makes it through a pregnancy depends not only on what you eat during your pregnancy but also on how well you've eaten for your entire lifetime.

The months immediately preceding a pregnancy are especially important for a healthy pregnancy. What you eat and how you take care of yourself before and during a pregnancy affects your health as well as your baby's. This means eating healthful, well-balanced meals with foods high in nutritional value. You also need to eat enough calories to create the right hormone balance for becoming pregnant. The more nutrient stores you have before getting pregnant, the faster you'll recuperate and get your body back into shape after delivery.

Extra Calories for Pregnancy

Once you're pregnant, the wheels of growth begin to turn. All the nutrient building blocks need to be in place to support the new growth of your body and your baby.

During your pregnancy, eat extra calories each day, since it takes about 80,000 calories throughout your nine-month term to develop your baby. That means roughly 320 extra calories a day, more if you're physically active. On average, you should eat a total of 2,200 to 2,400 calories a day.

A weight gain of 26 to 32 lb. during pregnancy is usually considered normal and healthy. Of this, about 20 lb. reflect changes in your own body weight. The average baby weighs about 7.5 lb. at birth. Fluid, placenta, and membranes account for the rest of your weight gain.

Pregnancy is not the time to restrict food or go on a reducing diet, since these put your baby at risk of being born with a low birth weight. Low birth weight is linked to infant mortality, chronic illness, and long-term developmental problems.

Part of a healthy pregnancy means gaining some fat weight. As your body prepares for breast feeding, it lays down fat to store the extra energy that will be used to make breast milk. One of the benefits of nursing is that this fat automatically melts off as your baby grows and requires more milk. If you don't nurse, you'll have to work the fat off the hard way—with lots of aerobic exercise.

Protein during Pregnancy

Pregnancy is a time of tissue building and increased red blood cell formation—processes that demand extra nutrients, particularly protein. You need extra protein during pregnancy to support the rapid tissue growth going on inside your body.

A large portion of your extra calories should come from protein—meats, poultry, fish, and nonmeat sources of protein such as legumes and grains. About 70 percent of all the protein you eat is used to build fetal and placental tissues, as well as those of your body. The RDA for protein during pregnancy is an additional 10 g over what you were eating prior to becoming pregnant.

Vitamins for a Successful Pregnancy

Folic Acid and Vitamin B$_{12}$

Two vitamins important for a successful pregnancy are folic acid and vitamin B$_{12}$. Folic acid (or folate) is a B-complex vitamin necessary for a host of functions in the body, including the synthesis of RNA and DNA—the genetic material responsible for cell division. During pregnancy, folic acid helps create red blood cells for the increased blood volume that you, the fetus, and the placenta require.

Because of folic acid's role in the production of genetic material and red blood cells, a deficiency can impair fetal development and lead to malformation. Adequate folic acid appears to protect against two common but serious defects afflicting newborns: spina bifida, in which the spine fails to fuse in a certain place, and anencephaly, in which the brain does not fully develop.

To work, folic acid requires the presence of vitamin B$_{12}$, a nutrient vital to healthy blood and a normal nervous system. The two vitamins act as partners in the manufacture of iron-carrying hemoglobin in red blood cells.

Deficiencies of either vitamin can create nutritional anemias. Folic acid deficiency leads to a condition called megoblastic anemia. In this anemia, red blood cells are enlarged, carry less hemoglobin, and have a short life span. As a result, less oxygen is available for the processes necessary for the growth of the fetus and the maternal tissues.

If you took oral contraceptives prior to conceiving, your folic acid levels may be low. It is suspected that oral contraceptives may interfere with the body's ability to utilize folic acid, which creates a potential hazard because a developing fetus needs folic acid early on.

A vitamin B_{12} deficiency can also produce megoblastic anemia. This deficiency is rare and affects only a small percentage of pregnant women, probably because vitamin B_{12} is found in all animal food. Pregnant women who follow a strict vegetarian diet, however, are candidates for vitamin B_{12} deficiency. Others at risk include people with an inherited inability to absorb the vitamin (a condition called pernicious anemia) and those on long-term antibiotic therapy. Though not common, a vitamin B_{12} deficiency can cause irreversible damage to the nervous system.

Folic acid and vitamin B_{12} deficiencies are easily preventable. Before and during pregnancy, foods rich in these vitamins should be included in your diet. The best sources of folic acid are dark green leafy vegetables. Whenever possible, these should be eaten fresh and raw because storage and cooking destroy as much as 80 percent of the vitamin. Lima beans, cauliflower, liver, meats, eggs, and nuts also supply folic acid.

Vitamin B_{12} is easier to obtain from the diet than folic acid is. By eating adequate amounts of meats, fish, and dairy products, you can take in a sufficient supply of vitamin B_{12}.

Folic Acid and Vitamin B_{12} Requirements during Pregnancy

Folic acid requirements are nearly tripled during pregnancy—from 50 to 100 µg a day to 150 to 300 µg a day. For the body to absorb adequate amounts of folate during pregnancy, the RDA is 800 µg a day.

You can also take a folic acid supplement of 200 to 400 µg every day before pregnancy and during your first trimester once you're pregnant. Check with your physician as to the advisability of supplementation.

Similarly, vitamin B_{12} requirements increase during pregnancy. The recommendation is 4 µg a day for a pregnant woman, as compared with 2.2 µg a day for a nonpregnant woman.

Other Important Vitamins

Your requirement for vitamin B_6 increases slightly during pregnancy, since this nutrient must be present for the production of red blood cells and genetic material. If you're frequently nauseous while pregnant, you may not be getting enough vitamin B_6, according to some studies. However, I think we need more research on this issue to see how it all shakes out. Using oral contraceptives prior to conceiving may increase your requirement for this nutrient.

The RDA for vitamin B_6 during pregnancy is 2.2 mg a day. Excellent sources of vitamin B_6 are meats and whole grains.

Small increases in the RDAs for pregnancy are suggested for vitamins D, E, C, thiamin, riboflavin, and niacin. As for vitamins A, K, and beta-carotene, there are no extra requirements. I strongly discourage megadosing of vitamins during pregnancy because many vitamins, including water-soluble vitamins, can be toxic to the developing baby. In fact, too much vitamin A has been linked to birth defects.

Minerals for a Successful Pregnancy

Calcium

Calcium is a construction material for the fetus, one that builds strong bones and teeth. It relies on phosphorus for normal skeletal formation and vitamin D for proper absorption. A well-balanced diet, fortified by ample amounts of calcium-rich foods, ensures proper absorption and utilization of calcium and contributes to a healthy outcome for you and your baby.

Calcium demands during pregnancy are high for two important reasons. First, greater amounts of the mineral are required for the calcification (hardening) of the fetus's developing bones and tooth buds. Second, your body stores more calcium during pregnancy to prepare for the greatly increased needs of this mineral for lactation.

For your body to absorb adequate amounts of calcium during pregnancy, the RDA is 1,200 mg a day, compared with 800 mg for a nonpregnant woman. This allowance is based on three factors: the amount of calcium you absorb, the amount taken in by the fetus, and the amount you excrete. Where a nonpregnant woman only absorbs about 10 to 20 percent of the calcium in food, a pregnant woman absorbs 40 percent.

You need a steady supply of adequate dietary calcium throughout your pregnancy. As the fetus develops, it needs more calcium. From the 1,200 mg in your diet, the fetus uses about 25 to 30 percent (360 mg a day), especially in the last trimester for skeletal growth. Additionally, calcium is stored in your bones for use during lactation.

Risks of a Calcium Deficiency

Both you and your baby suffer if the prenatal diet is short on calcium. A severe and prolonged calcium deficiency during pregnancy can result in poor development and abnormal calcification of the baby's bones and teeth. When intake is low, your bones may have to give up calcium to satisfy the baby's needs. This robs your stores of needed calcium, making additional calcium unavailable for lactation.

Another potential risk of low calcium intake is eclampsia (also called toxemia). This is a rare but serious complication that involves fluid retention, high blood pressure, loss of protein in the urine, and eventually convulsions and coma.

An additional reason to be concerned about calcium intake involves your health in later years. Frequent pregnancies combined with a long-standing calcium deficiency may contribute to osteoporosis.

Iron

While pregnant you need twice as much iron (30 mg daily). Iron demands increase during pregnancy because you must manufacture enough oxygen-carrying hemoglobin for yourself and your baby. Iron is also used to build red blood cells and replace blood lost during delivery.

In the first trimester of your pregnancy, the fetus accumulates most of the iron needed and will draw on your iron stores even if they're low. This can put you at risk of anemia unless you stock up on iron-rich foods like meats and dark green vegetables. But very few mothers-to-be get enough iron from food. That's why iron supplementation is usually recommended if you're pregnant. Always consult your obstetrician in matters regarding supplementation.

Sodium

Your body will retain fluid during pregnancy. This is normal and doesn't need to be treated with a sodium-restricted diet. A low-sodium diet stresses the body's fluid balance during pregnancy. But don't go overboard by eating a lot of salty foods. No more than 1 to 1.5 teaspoons of salt should be eaten daily.

Other Minerals

Requirements for several other major minerals go up during pregnancy. Magnesium is one of these, since it plays a key role in tissue growth. The pregnancy RDA for magnesium is 320 mg a day, compared with 280 mg a day for nonpregnant women. Good food sources include green vegetables, nuts, seeds, legumes, whole grains, and meats.

Phosphorus works together with calcium to maintain a specific ratio of one part phosphorus to two parts calcium in bone. This ratio is needed for both minerals to be used properly by the body. During pregnancy, you need 1,200 mg of phosphorus a day. Phosphorus-rich foods include meats, poultry, eggs, whole grains, seeds, and nuts.

We don't know much about the requirements for trace minerals during pregnancy, even though they're involved in growth and reproduction. The requirements for zinc, iodine, and selenium increase slightly during pregnancy, but if you eat a wide variety of food from all food groups, you're sure to get what you need in way of trace minerals.

Alcohol, Caffeine, and Artificial Sweeteners

Alcohol is a dangerous drug to use during pregnancy and has been associated with higher rates of miscarriage and low-birth-weight deliveries. It also can severely affect the baby through a syndrome called fetal alcohol syndrome (FAS). FAS causes growth retardation, heart defects, joint and limb problems, and arrested intellectual development. Alcohol should be eliminated or very limited in your diet.

The evidence about the effects of caffeine on babies is mixed, but several studies have shown evidence of birth defects. Researchers have recently observed that the amount of caffeine in 3 cups of coffee per day can decrease a woman's chance of becoming pregnant. Caffeine should also be eliminated or very limited in your diet.

Because you want to gain weight during pregnancy, there's no reason to use artificial sweeteners. Enjoy the benefits of being pregnant and use a little sugar, honey, or maple syrup for a change.

Contaminants in Foods

Many foods carry contaminants. Some are there naturally, some are caused by pollution. It's critical that you avoid foods that may contain contaminants because

Table 24-1

FOOD GUIDE FOR PREGNANT WOMEN

Food Groups	Daily Serving	Serving Size Examples
Milk and Milk Products		
(Supplies calcium, riboflavin, protein, vitamin B_{12}, vitamin A, and vitamin D)	4 servings daily (5 servings for adolescent mothers-to-be)	1 cup milk or yogurt 2 cups cottage cheese 1⅓ oz. cheese
Breads and Cereals		
(Supplies riboflavin, thiamin, niacin, iron, protein, magnesium, folic acid, and fiber)	6 to 11 servings a day, whole grain or enriched	1 slice bread ½ cup cooked cereal, rice, or pastas 1 oz. ready-to-eat cereal
Vegetables		
(Supplies vitamin A, beta-carotene, riboflavin, iron, magnesium, and fiber)	3 to 5 servings a day, green and yellow, starchy vegetables	½ cup cooked or chopped raw 1 cup leafy, raw
Fruits		
(Supplies vitamin A, vitamin C, and fiber)	2 to 4 servings a day, citrus fruits, melons, berries, and all others	1 whole fruit ½ cup juice ¼ melon ½ grapefruit ½ cup cooked/canned ¼ cup dried
Meat and Meat Alternatives		
(Supplies protein, phosphorus, vitamin B_6, vitamin B_{12}, niacin, thiamin, iron, zinc, and magnesium)	3 servings a day of lean meat, poultry, fish, shellfish, and vegetable protein sources	2 to 3 oz. lean, cooked 2 eggs 4 egg whites 1 cup cooked dried beans or peas 2 tbsp. peanut butter
Fats		
(Supplies vitamin A, and vitamin E)	3 to 6 servings a day, unsaturated vegetable oils, salad dressings, spreads, and nuts	1 tsp. spreads 1 tsp. vegetable oils 1 tbsp. salad dressing 1 oz. nuts
Sweets		
(Supplies energy)	Honey, maple sugar, sugar	Consume in moderation as needed for extra calories.
Water	8 or more glasses a day	

even traces can affect the health of your baby. To avoid lead contamination, fruit juice and acidic foods should be stored in glass or plastic containers. Don't use leaded crystal or ceramic containers. Tap water from older homes that might have lead pipes and faucets should be tested for lead content.

Large fish such as swordfish, shark, or marlin can be contaminated with mercury, so avoid these foods. Tuna intake should be limited to .5 lb. per week. Fresh fish can also be contaminated with pesticides and PCBs. Fish from the Great Lakes, the Hudson River, and freshwater fish from other inland waterways caught by recreational fishermen may be tainted with PCBs. Freshwater carp, wild catfish, lake trout, whitefish, bluefish, mackerel, and striped bass are the most likely to contain high PCB levels.

In general, pesticides and PCBs accumulate in fat. Always eat low-fat fish and meats, and trim the fat to avoid possible contamination.

Food Poisoning

Food poisoning by bacterial contamination can harm you and the baby. If you're traveling in foreign countries, don't buy food from street vendors, and eat only cooked foods, including fruits and vegetables. Use only boiled or bottled water, including the water used for ice cubes.

Soft cheeses like Brie and Camembert can be contaminated with a bacteria called listeria. Avoid eating these during your pregnancy.

Never eat raw animal foods while you're pregnant. They can contain parasites that will harm you and your baby. Avoid raw or unpasteurized milk, raw or undercooked shellfish, fish, eggs, poultry, or meat. Eat all meats well done. Don't eat foods that contain raw eggs, such as homemade eggnog, ice cream, Caesar salad dressing, raw cookie dough, or pancake batter.

Psychological Adjustments

After working so hard to get your body lean and fit, it may take some psychological adjustment to accept a pregnant body. You've worked hard to build your body. Now work on building your baby's body by eating more food to get all the nutrients you need. The food guide in table 24-1 can help you plan your meals for a healthy pregnancy.

It's critical to the health of your baby to give it all the energy and nutrients that it needs to grow healthy and strong. You have nine short months to give the baby the best start on life that it can have.

CHAPTER 25

High Performance through the Ages

Growing Older and Eating Smarter

There's a familiar saying about growing old gracefully. But wouldn't you rather grow old actively instead? It's clear that you can, by taking action now with things as simple as diet and exercise. With the health and vitality that come from making the right lifestyle choices, you *can* live an active lifetime—and perform strongly every minute of it. Following are some nutrition and exercise tips to help you be strong and active throughout every period of your life.

Ages Twenty to Thirty-Plus

Avoiding Weight Gain
One of my major concerns for people in this age group is the tendency to eat too much fast food, as well as highly processed convenience foods. These foods are too high in fat, which opens the door to weight gain. In fact, most weight gain among Americans occurs between the ages of twenty-five and thirty-four. That being the case, you must control the fat in your diet, eat a lot of carbohydrates, and keep your activity levels high with a combination of exercise and recreation. Yet don't go overboard. Many people, particularly young women, take dieting and exercise to extremes and fall prey to the eating disorders anorexia and bulimia. Both disorders are life-threatening and usually require intensive therapy and nutritional counseling to treat.

Weight gain also sets in because of physiological changes that begin taking place in your twenties and thirties. Beginning at age twenty, your aerobic function begins to decline. Unless you continue to train, that function will continue to drop off, and your fat-burning ability will be impeded.

Around age thirty, you start losing muscle mass—another factor that hinders weight control. With strength training, however, you can keep a much higher percentage of lean muscle and thus control your weight.

Watch Sodium

Fast foods and convenience foods are also high in sodium and low in potassium. An excess of sodium causes potassium to drain from the body, creating unhealthy imbalances, as well as fluid retention. My advice for curbing the use of fast foods is to try to cook at home more often, using easy-to-prepare foods such as those found in my cookbook *The High Performance Cookbook* (Macmillan). The recipes in it are designed specifically for people with busy, active lifestyles, as are the recipes found in the High-Performance Menu Plans in appendix A.

Early Protection against Osteoporosis

Women in this age group need to make sure they take in enough calcium to prevent bone loss later on in life. You can build up the amount of calcium in your bones until about age thirty, when the mineral content in bones reaches its peak. So the time to really concentrate on getting enough bone-building calcium is when you're in your twenties. That way, you can help protect yourself against osteoporosis.

Another excellent defense is to start exercising in your twenties or thirties to build up your bone density before age-related losses take their toll later. In a study at the University of California in San Francisco, sixty-three women ranging in age from twenty to thirty-five were randomly assigned to exercising and nonexercising groups. The exercisers did aerobics and weight training for an hour three times a week. All the women received calcium supplements or a placebo.

After two years, the exercisers had shored up their bone density in four places: the spine, the neck, thighs, and heels. Taking calcium supplements had no real effect, probably because the women were already eating a calcium-rich diet, according to the study. The point is, you can build bone early on with as little as three hours a week of exercise.

Iron Needs

In addition to calcium, women should be sure to get enough iron in the diet. These are the menstruating and childbearing years—two conditions in which the needs for iron are increased. If iron is in short supply, you risk becoming anemic. Anemia reduces the oxygen-carrying capacity of the blood, resulting in abnormal fatigue and lack of energy for activity or exercise. Bolster your body by eating iron-rich foods; combine them with vitamin C–packed foods to improve iron absorption.

Guidelines for Ages Twenty to Thirty-Plus

To sum up my recommendations:

- Stick to natural, nutrient-rich foods.
- Follow a high-carb, low-fat diet and exercise several times a week, including strength training.
- Don't diet obsessively.
- Cut down on sodium by limiting the convenience foods you eat.
- Make sure you're getting enough calcium and iron daily.

Ages Forty to Fifty-Plus

Watch Calories

In your forties and fifties, you generally have different nutritional needs than you did at twenty or thirty. Unless you're very active, you may need to restrict your calories somewhat to control your weight. But don't depend too much on fake sugars and fake fats to help you. These haven't been shown to help much with weight maintenance.

Another reason you may need fewer calories is loss of muscle tissue. If you have lost muscle tissue with age, your body can't burn up calories as well. But most people don't compensate. They eat more calories instead. Combined with a sedentary lifestyle, these extra calories turn into unwanted pounds. Before long, there's a big shift in body composition from less muscle to more body fat.

It's particularly important to watch fat intake not just to avoid weight gain, but to reduce the risk of heart disease and cancer. At the same time, be sure to eat foods of high nutritional value such as complex carbohydrates and lean proteins. These have a larger proportion of vitamins and minerals per calorie than processed foods. Wash your meals down with water too so that you stay well hydrated. In addition, eat lots of fresh fruits and vegetables, especially because they're full of disease-fighting phytochemicals.

Exercise Recovery

When you were in your twenties, your body could recover from a hard workout in as little as six hours. But by age forty, it now takes you forty-eight hours to recover. One reason is that aging makes your connective tissue—tendons, ligaments, and joint capsules—stiffer, less flexible, and less able to stand the wear and tear of exercise. Unless you take precautions, you're setting yourself up for injury.

The best preventive approach is to follow sound nutritional principles like those covered in this book. Eating properly can help speed up the recovery process and rebuild tissues that have broken down. The use of antioxidants from food and supplements is critical, too, since these nutrients help tissues recover better and regenerate more quickly following exercise.

Heart Health

More than ever, now's the time to control the fats and cholesterol in your diet. A high blood cholesterol level is one of the three major risk factors for heart disease, along with cigarette smoking and high blood pressure. Lowering blood cholesterol levels will significantly reduce your risk of heart disease. To do so, simply eat more low-fat foods, fruits, vegetables, and whole grains. As for animal proteins, choose smaller portions of foods like fish, poultry with the skin removed, and lean meats.

Along with cholesterol control, make sure you keep up an aerobic exercise program to bolster your cardiovascular health.

Nutrition and Cancer Protection

The relationship between diet and cancer is not as clear-cut as it is with heart disease. However, research does show that some foods increase or decrease your chances of developing certain kinds of cancer. In your forties and fifties, start heeding the following nutritional guidelines concerning cancer, although these should be followed by every age group:

✔ Maintain a healthy weight, since obesity is linked to increased death rates from some cancers, including breast, prostate, pancreatic, ovarian, colon, gall-bladder, and uterine.

✔ Keep your fat intake low—20 to 25 percent of your total calories. Some evidence exists tying high-fat diets to cancer.

✔ Fill up on fiber. Fiber keeps material moving through your system for good digestive health, and it appears to remove carcinogens from the body.

✔ Eat foods high in antioxidants and phytochemicals, since these seem to have a cancer-protective effect on the body.

✔ Limit your consumption of smoked and nitrite-cured meats. High incidences of esophageal and stomach cancers have been reported in populations who eat large amounts of these foods.

✔ Grill safely. When the fat from broiling, charring, or grilling foods drips or splatters onto the heat source, it may be transformed into potentially cancer-causing chemicals called PAHs (polycyclic aromatic hydrocarbons). These chemicals then can rise from the smoke and deposit onto the cooking food. If the food is charred, PAHs can form directly on the food itself. Smoking and browning of meats will also cause PAHs to form. Home-smoked meats may contain more PAHs than commercial foods treated with liquid smoke. My advice is to be moderate in your use of these cooking methods.

Preventing Diverticulosis

The risk of developing diverticulosis—small pouches that project outward from the wall of the colon—increases with age, especially past the age of fifty. When these pouches become inflamed or ruptured, the problem is called diverticulitis. Its symptoms include cramps, fever, and nausea. Often surgery is required to correct it.

Diverticular disease can be prevented by eating a high-fiber diet, including fresh fruits, legumes and vegetables, and whole grains. High-fiber supplements are helpful, too, but can cause bloating and gas in some people.

Bone Density and Strength Training

Somewhere around fifty years old, both men and women begin to lose some bone mineral as part of the aging process. This can lead to osteoporosis, which causes 1.3 million fractures a year. Of those who suffer hip fractures, 20 percent die within a year, and half of those who survive are never able to walk independently again.

As women go through menopause, calcium loss from the bones speeds up. This is because the hormone estrogen is required to deposit calcium in the bones and to keep it there. During menopause, women's estrogen production falls off, and it stays very low for the rest of their lives. So women are missing one of the key ingredients for maintaining bone structure.

One of the best antidotes for osteoporosis and weakening bones is strength training. Even in your fifty-plus years, exercise can help restore up to 5 percent of bone loss. In 1994 the results of a landmark study of postmenopausal women were published, showing for the first time that a single treatment—strength training—reduced risk factors for spine and hip fractures, which accompany osteoporosis. At the USDA Human Nutrition Research Center on Aging at Tufts University, women aged fifty to seventy worked out on exercise machines twice a week for a year. At the end of the study, they had built up their bones, increased their strength and muscle mass, and improved their balance.

Saving Lean Tissue

In this age group, you also start risking myoatrophy and the problems that go along with it, including loss of bone. This is another reason that it's vital to start a strength-training program. And don't think for a moment that it's dangerous to do if you're in your fifties. The abundance of research proves otherwise. At Tufts University, researchers have been able to triple muscle strength in older people. At one time, the team's oldest exerciser was a hundred years old!

In other studies, researchers have taken muscle biopsies and found that muscle tissue from older strength trainers looked like that of younger men—more proof that strength training turns back the aging clock.

Any exercise is dangerous if you jump into it after being sedentary all your life or if you have a preexisting medical condition that puts you at risk. Start an exercise program only with your doctor's blessing. Begin your program slowly, with short periods of activity performed under the guidance of a qualified exercise trainer.

Nutrition during Menopause

Menopause is the period of women's lives in which hormonal changes mark the end of the menstrual and reproductive years. Frequently, menopause brings with it emotional stress, irritability, and nervous symptoms. Though hormonal in nature, these symptoms can be greatly alleviated by a healthy, carb-rich diet and regular exercise.

Vitamin E has been used to treat the headaches and hot flashes associated with menopause. My recommendation would be to get the extra vitamin E needed by taking an antioxidant supplement.

If you're a woman past fifty, you may not need to worry as much about iron, which had been important during your childbearing years to rebuild blood components lost with menstruation.

During menopause and afterward, you should have 1,500 mg a day of calcium to help prevent or treat osteoporosis. Many doctors prescribe estrogen replacement therapy to prevent osteoporosis, and along with this therapy, calcium supplements. In addition, you should regularly strength train, since this has been proven to slow the loss of bone.

This period is also the time in a woman's life to start eating more soy foods. The phytoestrogens in them can help normalize estrogen levels. Menopausal women typically have low levels of estrogens, and these can be raised by phyto-estrogens.

Guidelines for Ages Forty to Fifty-Plus

My major recommendations include:

- Make sure you're eating the right number of calories each day to maintain a healthy weight and fuel your body for exercise and activity. Moderate your use of artificial sweeteners and fake fats.
- Watch your fat intake to protect yourself against fat-related diseases.
- Drink eight to ten glasses of water a day.
- Follow a high-fiber diet.
- Plan your diet around heart- and cancer-protective foods.
- Strength-train to build and preserve muscle and bone density.
- Make sure you're getting at least 1,500 mg a day of calcium from food and supplements if you're a woman.
- Include more soy foods in your diet.

Ages Sixty-Plus

Nutrient needs change abruptly and dramatically in this age group, especially since the older we get, the harder it is for our bodies to fully utilize certain key nutrients. What follows is some information on nutritional trouble spots to help you make vital adjustments in your nutrition as you get older.

Carbohydrates and Blood Sugar

With age, your glucose-processing mechanisms give way. Higher levels of sugar tend to float around in the blood, a condition that's stressful to the body and leads to blood sugar metabolism disorders like diabetes. Avoiding refined, sugar-loaded foods in favor of complex carbohydrates helps regulate blood sugar.

Also, eating plenty of complex carbs puts more fiber in the diet. Like a bouncer in a nightclub, fiber keeps the digestive tract running smoothly and throws out potential carcinogens before they can stick around to do any damage.

Fluids

The older you get, the more you must concentrate on drinking water as a part of your diet. In later years, thirst signals get short-circuited due to disturbances in the thirst mechanism. You're thirsty, but you don't know it. The risk of dehydration is high. Dehydration can lead to low blood pressure, elevated body temperature, nausea and vomiting, constipation, and low urine output.

There's more. Because the functioning of organ systems slows down a bit with age, it will take your body longer to get rid of toxins. If you don't drink enough fluid, your blood volume decreases and the toxins become more concentrated in the bloodstream. Many cases of dizziness and disorientation in the elderly are commonly due to dehydration. This is particularly critical if you take any medications. Even a normal dose can become toxic if you are slightly dehydrated.

To avoid these problems, drink at least 8 cups of fluid every day, not counting any caffeine-containing beverages. Always make sure to drink a cup of water before and after exercise. And if you're active in the heat, you need to drink even more.

Sodium

Limit your intake of sodium, since this mineral can aggravate high blood pressure. It's wise to cut your daily sodium intake to less than 3,000 mg by watching the amount of salt you use on your food. Instead of salt, experiment with herbs and nonsodium seasonings to enhance the flavor of your meals. Read labels carefully, too. Many canned, frozen, and fast foods are loaded with sodium.

Vitamin D

Unless retired to the Sunbelt, most Americans don't spend as much time outside as they once did, especially during the winter months. This lack of sun exposure, combined with a natural decrease in the body's ability to make its own vitamin D as we age, can make you more dependent on your diet to get enough vitamin D. As we've seen, vitamin D is essential for the absorption of calcium. Conveniently, many milk products, which are great sources of calcium, are fortified with vitamin D. Have at least two servings of them every day.

Nutrient Absorption

As many as 25 to 30 percent of people age sixty-five and 40 percent of eighty-year-olds suffer from *atrophic gastritis,* the inability to secrete enough stomach acid to kill off bacteria. The bacteria stays in the stomach and upper part of the small bowel, interfering with the absorption of calcium, folic acid, and vitamin B_{12}. This can lead to worrisome deficiencies. For example, inadequate calcium is risky for bone health. You want to guard against a short supply of folic acid, since it's now recognized as a protective nutrient, particularly against cervical cancer. An insufficiency of vitamin B_{12} can cause a buildup of homocysteine, a protein-like substance, in the tissues and blood. High homocysteine levels have been linked to heart disease.

If you think you suffer from atrophic gastritis, ask your physician about taking vitamin and mineral supplements.

Vitamin A

There's a growing consensus among many nutrition scientists that the RDA for vitamin A may be too high for people past age sixty. Their livers aren't able to clear nutrient as effectively, and it tends to build up in the system. This accumulation can be toxic. It may not be wise to supplement with extra vitamin A. Instead, rely on vitamin A–rich foods like carrots, yams, cantaloupes, and any yellow or orange vegetables.

B Vitamins

Not too long ago, it was learned that as many as three in ten people over age sixty-five may not be eating enough B vitamins, including folic acid, to prevent heart attacks and strokes. Researchers at the Human Nutrition Research Center on Aging at Tufts University studied 1,200 adults aged sixty and over and found that those who were deficient in B vitamins had high blood levels of homocysteine, a chemical linked to clogged arteries.

Eat Iron-Rich Foods

Iron-poor blood isn't the brainchild of iron supplement marketers; it's a bona fide health problem. As you age, you're at a greater risk of developing anemia, also known as iron deficiency. This occurs because there's a natural drop in hemoglobin, the oxygen-carrying protein particle in red blood cells. Most of the body's iron is found in hemoglobin. When hemoglobin declines, so does iron. The best defense is to make iron-wise food choices, including low-fat red meats. Combine iron-containing foods with vitamin C–rich foods, since vitamin C helps the body take up iron.

Immunity

You may be deficient in certain vitamins and minerals, and this is a threat to immunity. A study by the World Health Organization recruited ninety-six men and women over age sixty-five to see whether taking certain nutrients could bolster their immune function. Half the participants took a placebo, and the other half took a formulation containing eighteen vitamin and minerals—most at levels near the RDA. The study lasted twelve months, with two-week follow-ups throughout the year to see how many illnesses the participants had experienced.

After analyzing the data, the researchers found that the supplement users had far fewer infections and sick days during the year than those taking the placebo. Plus, lab tests confirmed improvements in immunity among those who took supplements.

Antioxidants and Aging

Some researchers think immunity is threatened by a lifelong buildup of oxidative damage to infection-fighting white blood cells. Antioxidants appear to counter this. In a study at the U.S. Department of Agriculture's Nutrition Research Center on Aging at Tufts University, researchers looked into the effect of vitamin E supplementation on the immune systems of healthy adults over age sixty. Taking 800 mg of vitamin E a day bolstered their immune systems.

With aging, enzyme activity drops off, and this decline can generate more free radicals. But one enzyme—catalase—doesn't appear to slow down. This special enzyme assists in the synthesis of protein in the body and has an interesting link to age-related muscle loss (myoatrophy). The older you get, the less protein your body makes. One consequence of this is muscle loss. Animal studies show that catalase activity actually increases with age, as if to exert some sort of protection against muscle loss. Coincidentally, animals with the highest catalase activity have the most muscle weight, meaning that catalase appears to preserve muscle in some way. Even more interesting is the fact that aging animals fed with antioxidants have more muscle than animals fed standard chow. These findings have motivated the researchers to investigate similar results in humans, and I suspect we'll see some intriguing data in the future.

Although it appears that deficiencies can be corrected by taking supplemental nutrients, it's far better to spruce up your diet by eating a variety of healthy foods, especially those rich in antioxidants. As an extra safeguard, I do recommend taking a daily antioxidant formula, but don't megadose on supplements.

Dental Health and Nutrition

Another cause of nutritional problems may be your teeth. If eating is painful or if you have poorly fitting dentures, you may be hurting your diet. Either way, your diet is compromised and so may be your nutritional health. Discuss these problems with your dentist.

Staying Strong

From the flick of your eyelid to the lifting of a heavy object, muscle powers your every action. Losing muscle means losing strength. What was once so easy to do—carrying grocery bags, picking up children, raking the yard—can become nearly impossible as muscle strength declines.

Loss of muscle strength is distressing because it impairs your mobility and limits your independence. The reason so many elderly fall and suffer debilitating fractures is primarily due to muscular weakness. In fact, falls are a leading cause of accidental death in people over age sixty-five.

Strength training has many positive effects on the health of people of all ages. And get this: The older you are, the more significant the impact. It's never too late to start, either.

Researchers at Tufts University studied the effects of strength training on ninety-year-old frail residents of a nursing home. Six women and four men (eighty-six to ninety-six years old) participated in a standard progressive strength-training program, three times a week for eight weeks. They had constant supervision, and their pulse rate and blood pressure were monitored during exercise.

The results were astounding. Attendance for all exercise sessions was nearly perfect. No one had any cardiovascular complications from the training. Muscle size increased, and strength improved 174 percent. Most important, the residents' day-to-day mobility improved significantly. The participants were walking 48 percent faster. Two people who had used canes prior to the study were able to walk unassisted. One person who initially couldn't get out of a chair without using his arms could do so on his own leg power.

Other similar studies have consistently shown that strength training helps you retain youthful strength. This form of exercise appears to be the only way to rebuild vital muscle tissue, regardless of how old you are. By that measure, it's a true fountain of youth.

Guidelines for Ages Sixty-Plus

In a nutshell, here are some rules to live well by:

- Include lots of complex carbs in your daily diet.
- Drink eight to ten glasses of water every day.

- Watch your sodium intake.
- Have two servings a day of vitamin D–fortified dairy products.
- Check with your doctor or dietitian about taking an antioxidant vitamin and mineral supplement daily.
- Include plenty of vitamin A–rich foods in your diet.
- Make sure you eat enough iron-rich foods each week.
- Work with your dentist to correct any dental problems that may be interfering with proper nutrition.
- Start a strength-training program with the blessing of your doctor.

Table 25-1

DETERMINE YOUR NUTRITIONAL HEALTH

Read the statements below. Circle the number in the yes column for those that apply to you or someone you know. Add the circled numbers to get your total nutritional score.

Nutrition Checklist	✓
• I have an illness or condition that made me change the kind and/or amount of food I eat.	2
• I eat fewer than two meals per day.	3
• I eat few fruits, vegetables, or milk products.	2
• I have three or more drinks of beer, liquor, or wine almost every day.	2
• I have tooth or mouth problems that make it hard for me to eat.	2
• I don't always have enough money to buy the food I need.	4
• I eat alone most of the time.	1
• I take three or more different prescribed or over-the-counter drugs a day.	1
• Without wanting to, I have lost or gained 10 lb. in the last six months.	2
• I am not always physically able to shop for, cook for, and/or feed myself.	2
Total Nutritional Score	

Total your nutritional score.

0–2 Good! Recheck your nutritional score in six months.

3–5 You are at moderate nutritional risk. See what can be done to improve your eating habits and lifestyle. Recheck your nutritional score in three months.

6–21 You are at high nutritional risk. Bring this checklist the next time you see your doctor, dietitian, or qualified health or social service professional. Talk with him or her about any problems you may have. Ask for help to improve your nutritional health.

Source: Reprinted with permission by the Nutrition Screening Initiative, a project of the American Academy of Family Physicians, the American Dietetic Association, and the National Council on Aging, Inc., and funded in part by a grant from Ross Products Division, Abbott Laboratories.

Nutritional Assessment at Any Age

Without good nutrition, you're putting your health on the line. To see whether you may be at risk for possible nutritional problems, take the Nutrition Screening Initiative (NSI) assessment in table 25-1. It's part of a project spearheaded by the American Academy of Family Physicians, The American Dietetic Association, and the National Council on Aging, Inc.

The assessment is a list of warning signs of poor nutritional health, similar to the warning signs used to assist in the early detection of cancer. How did you score? Recognizing and preventing health problems will help you extend your active lifetime, so you can achieve peak performance now—and in the future.

CHAPTER 26

Go for It

I hope you now have all the information you need for high-level performance and that you're ready to take action. Before you do, a few final thoughts:

✔ **Take this program one day at a time.** Even in a single day, the rewards of feeling better start rolling in—and continue to do so with each day, week, and month you stay true to a strong, high-performance lifestyle.

✔ **Keep moving, keep training, keep working out.** Your body, with its amazing system of muscles, joints, and bones, was meant to move. If the body doesn't move, its supporting structures like muscles and bones start *degenerating.* The exercising body, on the other hand, is *regenerating* itself, especially with the right nutrients providing the raw material for growth, maintenance, and lifelong health and vitality.

✔ **Use the diet and training logs in appendix E religiously.** It's a fact that when you write things down—and get in the habit of doing so—you're more likely to stick with your plan. Plus, you'll have a motivating record of your progress. Later on you can look back on it and see what worked best for you.

✔ **Don't go for gimmicks.** Every so often a new program or diet promising "health miracles without effort" comes along. Use some smarts to evaluate it: What are the credentials of the person or people behind it? What research backs it up? Is any component of nutrition or physical fitness left out? Is it something that can be continued for a lifetime?

✔ **Keep some perspective.** Every now and then, be sure to have some splurges. Your long-term results won't be affected by an occasional nutritional infringement.

✔ **Plan for rewards in your life.** We all need fun and joy in our lives. When you've achieved an important marker of any type—the addition of another mile or two to your running program, some lost pounds, or an important project finished because you had the energy to push on—plan something fun: an evening at your favorite restaurant, a weekend getaway, a new outfit, a gift for yourself.

✔ **Keep your eye on your ultimate goal,** whether it's to lose 10 lb., win your next race, or shave off points from your last cholesterol reading. Don't grumble about what you have to give up, because in reality all you're giving up is some bad habits you don't need in your life anyway. The payoff of a few small sacrifices is total fitness and well-being.

The main purpose of this book has been to teach you how to stay active, strong, and healthy. My hope is that you'll use it as a nutritional strategy for your life, starting now. As my work with athletes and exercisers has shown, and as recent research has proved, you can actually reinvent yourself. Energize yourself for everything you do. Develop lean muscle that is so universally attractive, and fundamentally healthy. Achieve your personal best in competition. Protect yourself against life-shortening diseases. Reverse physical evidences of aging like muscle loss and aerobic capacity.

What more could you ask for?

Now it's up to you. Go for it!

PART EIGHT

APPENDIXES

High Performance in Thirty Days: Putting Food Power into Practice

Like piecing together a jigsaw puzzle, planning a healthy diet takes some know-how and perseverance. You need more than forty different nutrients for good health, and no single food supplies them all. So how do you fit in all the nutrients you need to perform maximally?

My thirty-day menu plan does it for you. You can look ahead for the week and plan your shopping and your meals without worrying about the nutrition because it's already worked into the plan.

Based on the nutritional needs of physically active people, this plan offers 3,000 calories a day for men and 1,800 calories a day for women, with 65 percent from carbohydrates, 15 percent from protein, and 20 percent of the total calories from fat. Each day, you get exactly what you need from key food groups. For example:

- Bread, cereal, rice, and pasta group—6 to 11 servings
- Vegetable group—3 to 5 servings
- Fruit group—2 to 4 servings
- Milk group—2 to 3 servings
- Meat, poultry, fish, dry beans, eggs, and nuts group—2 to 3 servings
- Fats, oils, and sweets—used sparingly

On my thirty-day plan, serving sizes are based on the guidelines in table A-1.

Top Seventy Foods for Going Strong

My thirty-day menu plan, shown in table A-2, is designed around the top seventy foods needed for performing at a high level. They're foods fresh from the grocery store, packed with nutrients and phytochemicals that will make you healthy.

Table A-1

SERVING SIZE GUIDELINES FOR KEY FOOD GROUPS

Food Group	Serving Size
Bread, cereals, and other grains	1 slice bread; ½ cup cooked cereal, rice, or pasta; 1 ounce ready-to-eat cereal; ½ bun, bagel, or English muffin; 1 small roll, biscuit, or muffin; 3 to 4 small or 2 large crackers.
Vegetables	½ cup cooked or chopped raw vegetables; 1 cup raw, leafy vegetables; ½ cup cooked legumes; ¾ cup vegetable juice.
Fruit	1 medium piece of raw fruit, ½ grapefruit, 1 melon wedge, ½ cup berries, ½ cup diced cooked or canned fruit, ¼ cup dried fruit, ¾ cup of fruit juice.
Milk	1 cup skim milk or yogurt, 1½ oz. cheese, ½ cup of cottage cheese.
Meat, poultry, fish, and meat alternatives	3 oz. cooked lean meat, poultry, or fish (about the size of a deck of cards or the palm of a woman's hand). Other foods that count as 1 serving of meat include ½ cup cooked dry beans, 1 egg, 2 tbsp. of peanut butter, and 1 tbsp. of nuts or seeds.

Counting Nutrients

For the foods not mentioned in this book, you may find it helpful to purchase a pocket nutrient counter (the little guides sold at supermarket checkouts and in bookstores) to determine the grams of nutrients in specific foods. However, I realize it can be time-consuming to figure out the percentages of nutrients, weigh your foods, or count out grams of nutrients. Most of my clients don't want to bother with those calculations, either. So remember: Eat all the complex carbs you can—until you're blue in the face. There will be just enough room left over for the small amount of protein and fat you'll need for maximal performance.

Personalize the Plan

On this plan, you'll find full vegetarian days, partial vegetarian days, and good old-fashioned meat days, with room built in to personalize the plan and adapt it if you want to dine out. Use the information about restaurant and fast-food dining in chapter 19 to fill in your own favorites for designated meals. For example, if you know you'll be eating at a restaurant on Thursday night, but this meal doesn't show up on the menu until Friday, just switch the days on the calendar to meet your needs.

Most people eat nearly the same breakfast every workday. To break the monotony, I've included ten, one-minute breakfasts that are fast, simple, and easy to prepare. The same goes for dinner. On average, the American family has a repertoire of ten dinner meals, eaten day in and day out all year long. This menu plan builds on that concept, with ten different dinner suggestions rotated throughout the thirty-day menu plan, in addition to restaurant meals.

If you're strength training or cross training, you may need to eat more protein or carbs than the menus call for. If so, simply increase those nutrients to meet

Table A-2

TOP SEVENTY FOODS

Food Description	Serving	Calories	Carb. (g)	Protein (g)	Fat (g)	Cholest. (mg)
Breads and Cereals						
Bread, whole wheat	1 slice	61	12	3	trace	trace
Bagels, plain	1	200	38	7	2	0
English muffins, plain	1	140	27	5	1	0
Pita bread	whole	165	33	6	1	0
Crackers, graham, plain	1	55	10	1	1	0
Cookies, fig bars	2	100	21	1	2	11
Spaghetti, dry, enriched	2 oz. dry	211	43	7	trace	0
Rice, brown, cooked	½ cup	109	23	3	trace	0
Buckwheat groats, roasted, cooked	½ cup	284	62	10	2	0
Bulgur, cooked	½ cup	76	17	3	trace	0
Cereals, ready-to-eat, 40% bran flakes	1 cup	127	31	5	trace	0
Oats, dry	½ cup	303	52	13	5	0
Wheat germ, toasted, plain	1 oz.	108	14	8	3	0
Pancakes, buckwheat	1 4-in dia.	54	6	2	2	18
Vegetables						
Potato, baked with skin	1	220	51	5	trace	0
Yams, cooked (boiled and drained)	1 cup	158	38	2	trace	0
Parsnips, cooked (boiled and drained)	1 cup	130	31	2	trace	0
Carrot, raw	1	31	7	1	trace	0
Squash, winter, acorn, cooked	1 cup	115	30	2	trace	0
Corn, sweet, yellow, cooked	1 ear	83	19	3	1	0
Lettuce, cos or romaine	½ cup	5	1	1	trace	0
Spinach, raw	½ cup	6	1	1	trace	0
Broccoli, cooked (boiled and drained)	½ cup	22	4	2	trace	0

Table A-2 (continued)

Food Description	Serving	Calories	Carb. (g)	Protein (g)	Fat (g)	Cholest. (mg)
Tomatoes, red, ripe, raw	1	26	5	1	trace	0
Mushrooms, raw	1	5	1	1	trace	0
Fruits						
Apricots, dried, sulfured	10 halves	83	22	1	trace	0
Prunes, dried, uncooked	5	100	26	1	trace	0
Raisins, seedless	¼ cup	109	29	1	trace	0
Bananas, raw	1	105	27	1	trace	0
Oranges, raw	1	62	15	1	trace	0
Apples, raw, with skin	1	81	21	trace	trace	0
Strawberries, raw	1 cup	45	10	1	trace	0
Melon, cantaloupe, raw	½	93.45	22	2	trace	0
Orange juice, frozen, concentrate	1 cup	112	27	2	trace	0
Apple juice, canned or bottled	1 cup	117	29	trace	trace	0
Milk						
Milk, low-fat	1 cup	121	12	8	5	18
Milk, skim	1 cup	86	12	8	trace	4
Yogurt, coffee and vanilla	1 cup	194	31	11	3	11
Cheese, natural, cottage	½ cup	101	4	16	2	9
Cheese, natural, ricotta	½ cup	171	6	14	10	38
Cheese, natural, mozzarella	1 oz.	78	trace	8	5	15
Cheese, natural, Swiss	1 oz.	105	1	8	8	26
Protein Foods						
Eggs, whole, raw	1 large	75	trace	6	5	212
Eggs, white, raw	1 large	17	trace	4	0	0
Beans, black	½ cup	114	20	8	trace	0
Beans, navy	½ cup	129	24	8	trace	0
Beans, pinto	½ cup	116	22	7	trace	0
Soybeans, cooked	½ cup	149	9	14	8	0
Lentils, cooked	½ cup	115	20	9	trace	0
Peas, split	½ cup	116	21	8	trace	0

Table A-2 (continued)

Food Description	Serving	Calories	Carb. (g)	Protein (g)	Fat (g)	Cholest. (mg)
Tofu, raw, firm	½ cup	183	5	20	11	0
Seeds, sunflower	1 tbsp.	81	3	3	7	0
Seeds, sesame	1 tbsp.	47	trace	2	4	0
Peanuts, dry roasted	1 oz.	164	6	7	14	0
Peanut butter, chunky	2 tbsp.	188	7	8	16	0
Halibut, raw	3 oz.	94	0	18	2	27
Flounder, raw	3 oz.	77	0	16	1	40
Shrimp, raw	3 oz.	90	trace	17	1	129
Chicken, broilers or fryers, white, raw	½ breast	130	0	27	1	68
Chicken, broilers or fryers, dark, raw	1 leg	156	0	26	5	104
Turkey, light, raw	4 oz.	43	0	9	trace	23
Turkey, dark, raw	4 oz.	41	0	7	1	23
Beef, short loin, top sirloin, raw	4 oz.	141	0	24	4	69
Fats, Oils, and Sweets						
Oil, canola	1 tbsp.	124	0	0	14	0
Oil, olive	1 tbsp.	119	0	0	14	0
Oil, safflower	1 tbsp.	124	0	0	14	0
Frozen yogurt, 97% fat-free	3 oz.	90	18	2	1	0
Jams and preserves	1 tbsp.	55	14	0	0	0
Honey	1 tbsp.	65	17	0	0	0
Maple syrup	1 tbsp.	50	13	0	0	0

your exercise needs. This will automatically increase your calories as well. The beauty of these plans is that they can be used as a template to fit the nutrients you need to the exercise you're doing.

At first, use this menu as your bible. Once you get the hang of the number of servings and serving sizes you need to eat every day, you'll be able to vary the themes and further tailor the plan for your activity level and lifestyle.

Eat well, and enjoy.

Ten One-Minute Breakfasts

Each recipe is for 1 serving.

1. Aloha Muffin

1 multigrain English muffin
¼ cup cottage cheese or ricotta cheese
¼ cup crushed pineapple

Toast muffin. Spread with cheese and pineapple, and enjoy. 198 calories, 2 g of fat, 33 g of carbohydrate, 12 g of protein.

2. Old Reliable

1 cup bran cereal
1 cup low-fat milk
½ cup fresh berries

Mix together in a bowl and enjoy. 296 calories, 4 g of fat, 52 g of carbohydrate, 13 g of protein.

3. McBreakfast

3 fast-food pancakes with butter and syrup
1 cup orange juice
1 cup skim milk

723 calories, 15 g of fat, 128 g of carbohydrate, 19 g of protein.

4. Breakfast Pizza

1 whole wheat pita
¼ cup marinara sauce
1 oz. shredded part-skim milk mozzarella cheese
1 sliced mushroom

Spread marinara sauce on pita. Cover with cheese and mushroom slices. Broil or toast until cheese melts and bubbles. 275 calories, 7 g of fat, 38 g of carbohydrate, 15 g of protein.

5. Maple Oats

1 cup cooked rolled oats (the quick-cooking variety works great in the microwave)
½ tbsp. maple syrup
1 tbsp. honey-flavored wheat germ (I use Kletschmer's Honey Crunch.)

Mix together cooked oatmeal and maple syrup. Sprinkle with wheat germ. 223 calories, 3 g of fat, 40 g of carbohydrate, 9 g of protein.

6. Fast 'n' Easy, Too

1 cup low-fat vanilla yogurt
½ tbsp. natural crunchy peanut butter
3 tbsp. Grape-Nuts cereal

Mix together and crunch away! 407 calories, 7 g of fat, 68 g of carbohydrate, 18 g of protein.

7. Breakfast Dessert

½ cup skim milk
½ cup low-fat coffee yogurt
1 tbsp. chocolate syrup
¼ cup frozen unsweetened raspberries

Place all ingredients in blender and blend until smooth, about 45 to 60 seconds. 194 calories, 2 g of fat, 34 g of carbohydrate, 10 g of protein.

8. Apples 'n' Cheese

1 red apple, cored and sliced
1 oz. thinly sliced cheddar cheese
2 slices whole wheat toast

Place apples on bread and cover with cheese to make open-face sandwiches. Place under broiler or in toaster oven for 2 to 3 minutes or until cheese melts and bubbles. 331 calories, 11 g of fat, 45 g of carbohydrate, 13 g of protein.

9. Sweet Sunshine

2 tbsp. low-fat cream cheese
1 English muffin
½ banana, sliced lengthwise
1 tsp. brown sugar

Spread cream cheese on each muffin half. Cover cream cheese with banana slices and sprinkle with brown sugar. Place under broiler or in toaster oven for 1 to 2 minutes or until sugar melts and bubbles. 278 calories, 6 g of fat, 47 g of carbohydrate, 9 g of protein.

10. Metro Special

2 tbsp. low-fat cream cheese
1 bagel
1 tomato, sliced
½ cucumber, sliced
Dash of Vegesal or other vegetable seasoning salt

Spread cream cheese on bagel. Add tomato and cucumber slices. Sprinkle with Vegesal and close sandwich. 287 calories, 7 g of fat, 45 g of carbohydrate, 11 g of protein.

Ten Dynamite Dinners

1. Sesame Halibut

Preparation time: 20 minutes

½ lb. (8 oz.) halibut steaks (6 oz. for 1,800-calorie diet)
¼ tsp. sesame oil
2 tbsp. soy sauce
1 tsp. finely minced fresh gingerroot (one-half-inch slice)
1 clove garlic, finely minced
1 tsp. sesame seeds

1. Rinse the halibut with water and place on a broiler pan. Lightly brush the steaks with sesame oil.

2. Mix together the soy sauce, ginger, and garlic, and pour over the fish. Broil 10 minutes per inch. The steaks don't need to be turned.

3. Sprinkle the steaks with sesame seeds and return to the broiler for 30 seconds, until the seeds are golden brown. Watch closely; the seeds can burn very quickly.

Makes 2 servings. Each serving contains 148 calories, 4 g of fat, 3 g of carbohydrate, and 25 g of protein.

Note: This halibut goes great with the pineapple rice from the Grilled Honey Yogurt Chicken and Pineapple Rice recipe to come.

2. Phytochemical Delight (Fried Tofu Pocket with a Fruit Smoothie)

Preparation time: 20 minutes

8 oz. firm tofu, cut into ½-inch slices
2 tbsp. canola oil

½ tsp. ground ginger
½ tsp. garlic powder
¼ tsp. vegetable seasoning salt (I like Vegesal)
Pinch of freshly ground black pepper
1¼ tsp. soy sauce
2 large whole wheat pitas, cut in half
3 to 4 tbsp. barbecue sauce
2 thin slices raw onion
1 small tomato, sliced
1 cup alfalfa sprouts

1. Squeeze out excess water from the tofu into paper towels. Heat the canola oil in a nonstick skillet on medium-high for 30 to 45 seconds. Carefully place the tofu into the skillet. Fry for about 10 minutes on medium heat or until the cooked side is golden brown.

2. Flip the tofu and sprinkle with ground ginger, garlic powder, seasoning salt, and black pepper. Fry another 4 minutes or until the other side is browned.

3. During the last minute of frying, sprinkle the tofu with the soy sauce. Fry 30 seconds and flip. Fry another 30 seconds and remove from skillet. Don't let the oil smoke. Place the cooked tofu on a paper towel–lined plate.

4. Warm the pita in a toaster, but do not crisp. Spread inside pockets with barbecue sauce and place one fourth of the tofu into each pocket. Add onion, tomato, and alfalfa sprouts, and serve.

Makes 2 servings. Each serving contains 419 calories, 19 g of fat, 46 g of carbohydrate, 16 g of protein.

Fruit Smoothie

Preparation time: 5 minutes

2 cups skim milk
1 banana
1 cup frozen unsweetened strawberries
2 tsp. honey

1. Combine all ingredients in blender and blend for 1 minute or until smooth.

Makes 2 servings. Each serving contains 197 calories, 1 g of fat, 38 g of carbohydrate, 9 g of protein.

3. Spaghetti Carbonara

Preparation time: 15 minutes

6 oz. dry thin spaghetti (Ronzoni brand is excellent and easy to find)
2 oz. Canadian bacon

1 whole egg
2 egg whites
¼ tsp. freshly ground black pepper (or to taste)
4 tbsp. freshly grated Parmesan cheese

1. Cook pasta according to package directions. Meanwhile, chop the Canadian bacon into ¼-inch squares and grill in a nonstick skillet on medium-high heat for 3 to 4 minutes, stirring occasionally.

2. Beat together the whole egg and egg whites. Drain the cooked pasta and quickly return it to the cooking pot. While the pasta is still hot add the eggs, bacon, pepper, and Parmesan cheese. Toss well. The eggs will cook from the heat of the pasta, but remain creamy from the cheese. More fresh pepper can be added to suit your taste.

Makes 2 servings. Each serving contains 453 calories, 9 g of fat, 65 g of carbohydrate, 28 g of protein.

Note: A refrigerated egg substitute equivalent to two eggs may be used in place of the eggs.

4. *Asparagus and Shrimp Stir-Fry with Gingered Rice*

Preparation time: 40 minutes

½ cup long grain brown rice
1 cup boiled water
1 tbsp. candied (crystallized) ginger
2 tbsp. peanut oil
1 large clove garlic, minced
1 tsp. finely minced fresh gingerroot (one-half-inch slice)
10 oz. medium-sized shrimp, peeled and deveined, tails on (8 oz. for 1,800-calorie diet)
1 lb. thin asparagus, trimmed
1 cup sliced mushrooms (4 medium mushrooms)
1 tsp. cornstarch dissolved in 2 tbsp. soy sauce

1. Rinse the rice and toast it in a skillet over medium-high heat for about 6 minutes or until the rice begins to darken and pop. Carefully pour in boiling water, add the candied ginger, and stir. Lower the heat to simmer. Cover and cook for about 40 minutes or until all the water is absorbed and the rice is soft. Remove from heat and let steam another 5 minutes. Fluff with a fork before serving.

2. While the rice is cooking, heat the oil for 45 seconds on medium-high to high heat in a nonstick wok or skillet. Add half of the ginger and garlic and cook for 30 seconds. Add the shrimp and stir-fry for 2 to 3 minutes. Remove the shrimp with a slotted spoon to a bowl and set aside.

3. Add the rest of the ginger and garlic to the skillet and cook for 30 seconds. Add the asparagus and stir-fry for 1 minute. Add the mushrooms and stir-fry for another 3 minutes. Add the cooked shrimp and toss once. Lower the heat and add the cornstarch/soy sauce mixture. Toss to thicken. Serve over rice.

Makes 2 servings. Each serving contains 558 calories, 18 g of fat, 58 g of carbohydrate, 41 g of protein.

5. *Angelhair Scallops on a Spinach Bed*

Preparation time: 20 minutes

1 oz. sundried tomatoes, chopped
1 cup boiling water
10 large leaves fresh spinach, washed and stemmed (buy the prewashed spinach in a bag)
4 oz. dried angelhair pasta (I especially like lemon pepper pasta with this dish, but regular pasta is also good)
2 tbsp. olive oil
2 cloves garlic, finely chopped
½ lb. (8 oz.) bay scallops (6 oz. for 1,800-calorie diet)
2 lemon wedges
Pinch of freshly ground black pepper
2 tbsp. Parmesan cheese

1. Soak sundried tomatoes in boiling water for at least 10 minutes to soften. Arrange spinach leaves in a bed on two plates. Cook and drain pasta according to package directions.

2. While pasta is cooking, heat the oil in a large nonstick skillet for 30 seconds on medium high heat. Sauté the garlic and tomatoes for 1 to 2 minutes. Add the scallops and sauté one more minute. Remove from heat and toss in the noodles.

3. Serve warm on top of spinach beds. Sprinkle with lemon juice, black pepper, and Parmesan cheese just before serving.

Makes 2 servings. Each serving contains 509 calories, 17 g of fat, 56 g of carbohydrate, 33 g of protein.

Note: 10 oz. of peeled and deveined shrimp can be substituted for the bay scallops. Sauté until shrimp is pink and curled.

6. *Curried Rice and Lentils*

Preparation time: 40 minutes

½ cup raw lentils, cleaned and washed
1 cup water
¼ cup chopped onion

¼ cup thinly sliced celery
1 tbsp. curry powder
2 tbsp. butter
1 cup long grain rice
2 cups chicken broth (or one 14.4-oz. can)
⅔ cup raisins
¼ tsp. salt
½ cup coarsely chopped cashews

1. Place the lentils and water in a pot and bring to a boil. Lower heat and simmer for 30 minutes. Drain any excess water.

2. While the lentils are cooking, sauté the onion, celery, and curry powder in the butter in a 2-qt. saucepan until the celery is tender. Add the rice. Stir in the chicken broth, raisins, and salt. Cover pan and bring to boiling. Reduce heat; cover and simmer 15 minutes or until rice is done. Let stand, covered, for 10 minutes. Just before serving stir in the lentils and chopped cashews. Toss lightly to mix.

Makes 4 servings and is great as a leftover, hot or cold. Each serving contains 507 calories, 15 g of fat, 78 g of carbohydrate, 15 g of protein.

7. *Grilled Honey Yogurt Chicken with Pineapple Rice*

Preparation time: 45 minutes

¾ cup chicken broth
¼ cup pineapple juice from canned pineapple
½ cup long grain brown rice
½ cup plain nonfat yogurt
1 tbsp. honey
Pinch of salt and pepper
2 skinless, boneless chicken breast halves
4 canned pineapple rings

1. Preheat grill. Boil chicken broth and pineapple juice in a small saucepan. Add the rice and stir once. Cover, lower the heat, and simmer for 40 minutes or until all the water is absorbed and the rice is soft.

2. Meanwhile, stir together the yogurt, honey, salt, and pepper. Coat the chicken with the yogurt sauce and place on heated, closed grill for 20 minutes, turning once after 10 to 12 minutes.

3. Place the 4 pineapple rings on the grill during the last 5 minutes of cooking. Turn once. Chop 2 of the rings into chunks and toss into the rice before serving. Serve the other 2 rings on top of the chicken breasts, on a bed of rice.

Makes 2 servings. Each serving contains 455 calories, 3 g of fat, 72 g of carbohydrate, 35 g of protein.

Note: You can also serve this Indian-style chicken with leftovers of the curried rice in place of the pineapple rice. And if you have leftover chicken, it makes a great cold grilled chicken sandwich or salad for tomorrow's lunch.

8. *Pasta con Cioppino*

Preparation time: 30 minutes

1 tbsp. plus 1 tsp. olive oil
1 clove garlic, chopped
2 oz. raw mushrooms, sliced
½ tbsp. fresh chopped basil
½ tsp. fines herbs
Salt and freshly ground pepper to taste
2 tbsp. dry white wine
½ cup your favorite bottled marinara sauce
6 large mussels, washed and debearded (4 for 1,800-calorie diet)
6 littleneck clams (4 for 1,800-calorie diet)
8 medium shrimp, peeled and deveined (6 for 1,800-calorie diet)
1 tbsp. chopped fresh parsley
1 tsp. sweet butter (aka unsalted butter)
8 oz. dried penne pasta, or other tubular pasta such as ziti or rigatoni
2 fresh parsley sprigs

1. Boil water for pasta according to package directions. Heat the oil on medium high in a large nonstick sauté pan for 1 minute. Add the chopped garlic and heat for 30 seconds. Add the mushrooms and sauté for 2 minutes.

2. Add the basil, fines herbs, salt, and pepper. Flame with white wine (flaming is optional). Add the marinara sauce, mussels, clams, shrimp, parsley, and butter. Cover and simmer for 5 minutes or until the clams and mussels open.

3. While the shellfish is cooking, boil the pasta and drain in a colander. Distribute half the pasta on each plate and spoon the cioppino mixture evenly over the pasta. Garnish with parsley and serve.

Makes 2 servings. Each serving contains 631 calories, 15 g of fat, 96 g of carbohydrate, 28 g of protein.

9. *Sig's Slaw*

Preparation time: 25 minutes

2 oz. dried mung bean thread, cellophane noodles, or rice sticks
½ medium head of savoy cabbage (or green cabbage)
2 large carrots
8 oz. crabmeat, fresh or frozen and thawed (6 oz. for 1,800 calorie diet)

2 tbsp. canola oil
3 tbsp. rice vinegar
1 tbsp. low-sodium soy sauce
1½ tbsp. sugar
½ tsp. garlic powder
¼ tsp. salt
Dash of freshly ground black pepper
1 tbsp. toasted sesame seeds

1. Break the cellophane noodles into smaller threads and boil for 1 minute. Drain and rinse in cold water. Chop cabbage into squares and use a vegetable peeler to shred the whole carrots to make carrot curls, rather than slicing or chopping. Place in a large salad bowl. Add cellophane noodles and toss to mix.

2. In a small bowl or carafe mix the oil, vinegar, soy sauce, sugar, garlic powder, salt, and pepper. Pour over slaw and mix well. Add crabmeat and toss lightly again. Sprinkle with sesame seeds before serving.

Makes 2 servings. Each serving contains 684 calories, 20 g of fat, 98 g of carbohydrate, 28 g of protein.

10. *Easy Beans 'n' Rice*

Preparation time: 40 minutes (for the rice)

1 cup brown rice
1 cup canned chicken broth
1 cup water
1 15-oz. can black beans
1 15-oz. can diced tomatoes
4 tbsp. diced onion
2 tsp. chopped fresh cilantro
¼ tsp. chili powder
⅛ tsp. cumin
4 tbsp. low-fat sour cream
3 tbsp. chopped scallions (optional)

1. Bring the water and chicken broth to a boil in a saucepan and add the rice. Stir; cover and simmer about 40 minutes or until all the water is absorbed.

2. In a medium saucepan mix together the beans, tomatoes, onion, cilantro, chili powder, and cumin. Bring to a boil over medium high heat. Reduce heat to low, cover, and simmer for 5 minutes, stirring once or twice.

3. Serve beans over rice with a dollop of sour cream and a sprinkling of scallions.

Makes 2 servings. Each serving contains 642 calories, 6 g of fat, 120 g of carbohydrate, 27 g of protein.

Thirty-Day Menu—3,000 Calories

Day 1: Sunday

Breakfast

1 cup orange juice
4 slices French toast
3 tbsp. maple syrup
1 cup low-fat milk
1 cup coffee

Out for a Country Bike Tour or Picnic

Drink lots of water.

Packed Lunch on the Road

Swiss cheese sandwich on hearty whole wheat
    bread with 2 slices of cheese
Carrot and celery sticks
1 apple
2 Nature Valley Granola Bars (1 package)
1 box (8 oz.) sports drink

Packed Afternoon Snack

1 box (8 oz.) sports drink
¼ cup dried apricots
8 graham cracker squares

Dinner

Grilled Honey Yogurt Chicken (½ breast)
1 large bowl tossed salad
2 tbsp. salad dressing
1 cup pineapple rice
1 cup cooked broccoli
1 tsp. butter or margarine
2 slices crispy French bread
1 cup frozen yogurt topped with fresh straw-
    berries
Cranberry juice seltzer spritzer: ½ cup cran-
    berry juice mixed with soda water

Day 2: Monday

Breakfast

1 Aloha Muffin
1 cup low-fat milk
½ cup orange juice

Brown Bag Lunch

1 cup fruit yogurt
3 large squares Seasoned Ry-Krisp crackers
Green pepper and cucumber slices
1 cup fruit juice

Afternoon Snack

3 oz. or 1½ cups pretzels
2 tbsp. dry roasted peanuts
12-oz. can soda pop

Dinner

Asparagus and Shrimp Stir-Fry
2 cups gingered rice
Small tossed salad
1 tbsp. salad dressing
½ cup fruit sorbet
1 cup low-fat milk
4 small oatmeal raisin cookies

Day 3: Tuesday

Breakfast

Maple Oats
1 bagel
1 tbsp. cream cheese
1 cup low-fat milk
1 cup orange juice

Lunch

Mexican restaurant/fast food
1 bean burrito

1 cup rice
Tossed salad
1 tbsp. salad dressing
1 cup soft-serve ice milk

Afternoon Snack

1 cup fruit yogurt
3 tbsp. honey roasted peanuts
1 cup vegetable juice

Dinner

Pasta con Cioppino
1 slice Italian garlic bread
1 cup steamed zucchini and mushrooms sprin-
    kled with Parmesan cheese
1 cup low-fat milk
1 cup sherbet

Day 4: Wednesday
Breakfast

Fast 'n' Easy, Too
½ cup orange juice

Brown Bag Lunch

Turkey and Swiss cheese sandwich on hearty
    whole wheat bread with 1 slice of turkey
    and 1 slice of cheese
Carrot and celery sticks
1 pear
2 Nature Valley Granola Bars (1 package)
1 cup fruit juice

Afternoon Snack

3 cups microwave popcorn
12-oz. can soda pop

Dinner

Sesame Halibut
Large tossed salad
2 tbsp. light salad dressing
1 large baked sweet potato
1 corn on the cob

3 slices whole grain bread
2 tsp. butter or margarine
1 cup low-fat milk
½ cup frozen yogurt
4 small oatmeal raisin cookies

Day 5: Thursday
Breakfast

Sweet Sunshine
1 cup low-fat milk

Lunch

3 slices pizza with cheese
Large tossed salad
2 tbsp. light salad dressing
2 slices garlic bread
1 cup low-fat milk

Afternoon Snack

1 apple
6 graham crackers
1 cup low-fat milk

Dinner

Easy Beans 'n' Rice
Tossed salad
2 tbsp. light salad dressing
1 cup sorbet with fresh raspberries
2 small (1 oz. total) peppermint patties

Day 6: Friday
Breakfast

Old Reliable
1 raisin English muffin, toasted
1 cup orange juice

Brown Bag Lunch

Peanut butter and jelly sandwich on whole
    wheat
1 apple

Green and red pepper slices
1 cup low-fat milk

Afternoon Snack

1 cup fruit yogurt
3 oz. pretzels

Dinner

Enjoy a restaurant meal complete with
dessert.

Day 7: Saturday
Breakfast

Breakfast Dessert
Cinnamon-raisin bagel
1 tbsp. cream cheese

Lunch

Leftover Easy Beans 'n' Rice from Thursday
night dinner
1 cup low-fat milk
Frozen fruit juice bar

Afternoon Snack

6 Fig Newtons
½ cup grapes

Dinner

Spaghetti Carbonara
Large tossed salad with shredded mozzarella
2 tbsp. salad dressing
2 slices garlic bread
½ cup frozen vanilla yogurt with peanuts and
chocolate sauce

Day 8: Sunday
Breakfast

6 pancakes
2 tbsp. maple syrup
1 cup low-fat milk
1 cup orange juice

Out for a Country Bike Tour or Picnic

Drink lots of water.

Packed Lunch on the Road

Peanut butter and apple butter on hearty
whole wheat bread with 2 tbsp. peanut butter and 2 tbsp. apple butter
Carrot and celery sticks
1 apple
2 Nature Valley Granola Bars (1 package)
1 box (8 oz.) sports drink

Packed Afternoon Snack

1 box (8 oz.) sports drink
¼ cup dried apricots
8 graham cracker squares

Dinner

Enjoy a high-carbohydrate restaurant dinner.

Day 9: Monday
Breakfast

Breakfast Pizza
1 cup low-fat milk

Brown Bag Lunch

1 cup fruit yogurt
3 large squares Seasoned Ry-Krisp crackers
Handful of cherry tomatoes and cucumber
slices
1 cup fruit juice

Afternoon Snack

4 oatmeal cookies
1 cup milk

Dinner

Fried Tofu Pocket
1 cup brown rice
Large tossed salad
2 tbsp. light salad dressing
Fruit Smoothie

Day 10: Tuesday
Breakfast
Metro Special
1 cup low-fat milk

Lunch
Your best fast-food bet (see chapter 19 for a list)

Afternoon Snack
1 cup fruit yogurt
3 oz. pretzels

Dinner
Sig's Slaw
2 slices garlic bread
1 corn on the cob
Small tossed salad
Fat-free salad dressing
1 cup low-fat milk
1 cup fruit sorbet

Day 11: Wednesday
Breakfast
Old Reliable
1 cup orange juice

Brown Bag Lunch
Leftover Sig's Slaw
1 apple
1 pear
1 cup vegetable juice

Afternoon Snack
6 Fig Newtons
1 cup low-fat milk

Dinner
Sesame Halibut
Large tossed salad
2 tbsp. salad dressing

1 large baked potato
3 slices whole grain bread
2 tsp. butter or margarine
1 cup low-fat milk
1 cup fruit sorbet

Day 12: Thursday
Breakfast
McBreakfast

Lunch
Enjoy an ethnic vegetarian restaurant delight.

Afternoon Snack
½ bag low-fat microwave popcorn
½ cup grapes
12-oz. soda pop

Dinner
Curried Rice and Lentils
Tossed salad
2 tbsp. light salad dressing
1 cup frozen yogurt

Day 13: Friday
Breakfast
Apples 'n' Cheese
1 cup orange juice
1 cup low-fat milk

Brown Bag Lunch
Leftover Curried Rice and Lentils from last night's dinner
1 cup applesauce snack pack (2 packages)
1 cup vegetable juice

Afternoon Snack
3 oz. or 1½ cups pretzels
2 tbsp. dry roasted peanuts
12-oz. can soda pop

Dinner

High-carbohydrate restaurant dinner and pop-corn (popped in a healthy oil) at the movies.

Day 14: Saturday
Breakfast

1 Aloha Muffin
1 cup low-fat milk
1 cup cranberry juice

Lunch

1 cup bean soup
3 slices hearty whole wheat bread
Tossed salad
1 tbsp. salad dressing
1 apple
1 cup low-fat milk

Afternoon Snack

1 cup fruit yogurt
1 large square Seasoned Ry-Krisp cracker

Dinner

Enjoy a restaurant dinner complete with dessert.

Day 15: Sunday
Breakfast

1 cup orange juice
4 slices French toast
3 tbsp. maple syrup
1 cup low-fat milk
1 cup coffee

Out for a Hike

Drink lots of water.

Packed Lunch on the Road

Swiss cheese sandwich on hearty whole wheat bread with 2 slices of cheese

Carrot and celery sticks
1 apple
2 Nature Valley Granola Bars (1 package)
1 box (8 oz.) sports drink

Packed Afternoon Snack

1 box (8 oz.) sports drink
¼ cup dried apricots
8 graham cracker squares

Dinner

Sesame Halibut
1 large bowl tossed salad
2 tbsp. salad dressing
1 large baked potato
1 tsp. butter or margarine
1 cup cooked broccoli (prepare 2 cups, with 1 cup for tomorrow's lunch)
2 large squares corn bread
1 cup frozen yogurt topped with fresh straw-berries
Cranberry juice seltzer spritzer: ½ cup cran-berry juice mixed with soda water

Day 16: Monday
Breakfast

Maple Oats
½ cup orange juice
1 cup low-fat milk

Lunch

1 cup fruit yogurt
3 large squares corn bread from last night
1 cup cold cooked broccoli from last night with 1 tbsp. Italian dressing
1 pear
12 oz. soda pop

Afternoon Snack

2 Nature Valley Granola Bars (1 package)
1 cup low-fat milk

Dinner

Asparagus and Shrimp Stir-Fry
2 cups gingered rice
Small tossed salad
2 tbsp. salad dressing
1 roll
6 Fig Newtons
1 frozen fruit juice bar

Day 17: Tuesday

Breakfast

Sweet Sunshine
1 cup low-fat milk

Lunch

Mexican restaurant/fast food
1 bean burrito
2 cups rice
Tossed salad
1 tbsp. salad dressing
1 cup soft-serve ice milk

Afternoon Snack

1 cup fruit yogurt
3 tbsp. honey roasted peanuts
1 cup vegetable juice

Dinner

Pasta con Cioppino
3 slices Italian garlic bread
1 cup steamed vegetables
1 cup low-fat milk
1 cup fruit sorbet

Day 18: Wednesday

Breakfast

Breakfast Dessert
1 bagel
1 tbsp. fruit jam

Brown Bag Lunch

1 cup last night's leftover Pasta con Cioppino
  heated in a microwave
Carrot and celery sticks
1 apple
1 cup vegetable juice

Afternoon Snack

4 Fig Newtons
½ cup raisin and nut mixture

Dinner

Angelhair Scallops on a Spinach Bed
1 corn on the cob
2 rolls
1 cup low-fat milk
½ cup frozen yogurt with fruit syrup
4 graham cracker squares

Day 19: Thursday

Breakfast

Old Reliable
1 cup orange juice

Lunch

Your best fast-food bet (see chapter 19 for a
  list)

Afternoon Snack

1 cup fruit yogurt
2 large squares Seasoned Ry-Krisp crackers

Dinner

Sig's Slaw
2 hearty rolls
1 corn on the cob
1 cup low-fat milk
1 cup fruit sorbet

Day 20: Friday
Breakfast
Fast 'n' Easy, Too

Brown Bag Lunch
Turkey and Swiss cheese sandwich on hearty
   whole wheat bread with 2 slices of turkey
   and 1 slice of cheese
Carrot and celery sticks
1 pear
2 Nature Valley Granola Bars (1 package)
1 cup fruit juice

Afternoon Snack
3 oz. pretzels
1 cup vegetable juice

Dinner
Easy Beans 'n' Rice
Large tossed salad
Fat-free salad dressing
1 cup low-fat milk
1 cup sherbet with fresh berries
4 small (2 oz. total) peppermint patties

Day 21: Saturday
Breakfast
Metro Special
1 cup low-fat milk

Lunch
Large whole wheat pita stuffed with 2 slices
   cheese and lots of fresh veggies
3 oz. pretzels
2 frozen fruit juice bars
1 cup vegetable juice

Afternoon Snack
1 cup fruit yogurt
½ bagel

1 tbsp. peanut butter
1 tbsp. fruit jam

Dinner
Enjoy a restaurant dinner complete with
   dessert.

Day 22: Sunday
Breakfast
6 pancakes
2 tbsp. maple syrup
1 cup low-fat milk
1 cup orange juice

Out for a Country Bike Tour or Picnic
Drink lots of water.

Packed Lunch on the Road
Peanut butter and apple butter on hearty
   whole wheat bread with 2 tbsp. peanut butter and 2 tbsp. apple butter
Carrot and celery sticks
1 apple
2 Nature Valley Granola Bars (1 package)
1 box (8 oz.) sports drink

Packed Afternoon Snack
1 box (8 oz.) sports drink
¼ cup dried apricots
8 graham cracker squares

Dinner
Grilled Honey Yogurt Chicken (½ breast)
1 large bowl tossed salad
2 tbsp. fat-free salad dressing
1 cup pineapple rice
1 tsp. butter or margarine
1 cup cooked broccoli
2 slices crispy french bread
1 cup frozen yogurt topped with fresh berries
2 (1 oz. total) small peppermint patties

Day 23: Monday
Breakfast
McBreakfast

Brown Bag Lunch
1 leg quarter cold grilled chicken from last
    night's dinner
Green pepper and cucumber slices
2 large squares Seasoned Ry-Krisp crackers
1 cup (2 packages) applesauce snack pack
1 cup low-fat milk

Afternoon Snack
1 cup fruit yogurt
2 Fig Newtons

Dinner
Sig's Slaw
2 hearty rolls
1 corn on the cob
2 oatmeal raisin cookies
1 cup fruit sorbet

Day 24: Tuesday
Breakfast
Breakfast Pizza

Lunch
Enjoy an ethnic vegetarian restaurant delight.

Afternoon Snack
3 cups microwave popcorn
1 cup fruit juice
1 apple

Dinner
Sesame Halibut
Small tossed salad
1 tbsp. light salad dressing
1 large baked sweet potato
1 corn on the cob

3 slices whole grain bread
2 tsp. butter or margarine
1 cup low-fat milk
1 cup frozen yogurt with fruit syrup
4 small oatmeal raisin cookies
Cranberry juice seltzer spritzer: 1 cup cran-
    berry juice mixed with soda water

Day 25: Wednesday
Breakfast
Maple Oats
1 bagel
1 tbsp. fruit jam
1 cup low-fat milk

Brown Bag Lunch
1 cup fruit yogurt
2 large squares Seasoned Ry-Krisp crackers
Handful of cherry tomatoes and cucumber
    slices
1 cup fruit juice

Afternoon Snack
3 oz. pretzels
2 tbsp. honey roasted peanuts
1 cup vegetable juice

Dinner
Fried Tofu Pocket
1 cup brown rice
Small tossed salad
2 tbsp. fat-free salad dressing
½ cup frozen yogurt with fruit syrup
2 (1 oz. total) small peppermint patties

Day 26: Thursday
Breakfast
Old Reliable
1 bagel
1 tbsp. fruit jam
½ cup orange juice

Lunch

Your best fast-food bet (see chapter 19 for a list)

Afternoon Snack

6 Fig Newtons
1 cup low-fat milk

Dinner

Easy Beans 'n' Rice
Tossed salad
2 tbsp. light salad dressing
1 cup sorbet with fresh raspberries
2 small (1 oz. total) peppermint patties

Day 27: Friday
Breakfast

Sweet Sunshine
1 cup low-fat milk

Brown Bag Lunch

Peanut butter and jelly sandwich on whole
    wheat
1 apple
Green and red pepper slices
1 cup low-fat milk

Afternoon Snack

1 cup fruit yogurt
½ cup grapes
6 graham cracker squares

Dinner

Enjoy a high-carbohydrate restaurant meal.

Day 28: Saturday
Breakfast

Breakfast Dessert
1 English muffin
1 tbsp. fruit jam

Lunch

1 cup bean soup
3 slices hearty whole wheat bread
Tossed salad
1 tbsp. salad dressing
1 apple
1 cup low-fat milk

Afternoon Snack

1 cup fruit yogurt
2 large squares Seasoned Ry-Krisp crackers
1 cup vegetable juice

Dinner

Enjoy a night on the town complete with
    dessert.

Day 29: Sunday
Breakfast

1 cup orange juice
4 slices French toast
3 tbsp. maple syrup
1 cup low-fat milk
1 cup coffee

Out for a Hike

Drink lots of water.

Packed Lunch on the Road

Swiss cheese sandwich on hearty whole
    wheat bread with 2 slices of cheese
Carrot and celery sticks
1 apple
2 Nature Valley Granola Bars (1 package)
1 box (8 oz.) sports drink

Packed Afternoon Snack

1 box (8 oz.) sports drink
¼ cup dried apricots
8 graham cracker squares

Dinner

Angelhair Scallops on a Spinach Bed
1 large baked sweet potato
1 large square corn bread
1 cup frozen yogurt topped with fresh straw-
    berries
Cranberry juice seltzer spritzer: ½ cup cran-
    berry juice mixed with soda water

Day 30: Monday
Breakfast

Fast 'n' Easy, Too

Lunch

½ of 10-in. pizza with ground beef

Thirty-Day Menu—1,800 Calories

Day 1: Sunday
Breakfast

½ cup orange juice
2 slices French toast
1 tbsp. maple syrup
1 cup skim milk
1 cup coffee

Out for a Country Bike Tour

Drink lots of water.

Packed Lunch on the Road

Swiss cheese sandwich on hearty whole wheat
    bread with 1 oz. of cheese
Carrot sticks
1 apple
2 Nature Valley Granola Bars (1 package)

Packed Afternoon Snack

¼ cup dried apricots
6 graham cracker squares

Small tossed salad
1 tbsp. salad dressing
1 cup cranberry juice

Afternoon Snack

1 cup fruit yogurt
2 large squares Seasoned Ry-Krisp crackers
12-oz. soda pop

Dinner

Curried Rice and Lentils
1 roll
Tossed salad
2 tbsp. light salad dressing
½ cup frozen yogurt with fresh berries
2 (1 oz. total) small peppermint patties

Dinner

Grilled Honey Yogurt Chicken (½ breast)
1 tossed salad
2 tbsp. salad dressing
½ cup pineapple rice
1 cup cooked broccoli
1 tsp. butter or margarine
1 slice crispy French bread
1 cup frozen yogurt topped with fresh straw-
    berries

Day 2: Monday
Breakfast

1 Aloha Muffin
1 cup skim milk
½ cup orange juice

Brown Bag Lunch

1 cup fruit yogurt
2 large squares Seasoned Ry-Krisp crackers
Green pepper slices

Afternoon Snack

3 oz. or 1½ cups pretzels
2 tbsp. dry roasted peanuts

Dinner

Asparagus and Shrimp Stir-Fry
1 cup gingered rice
Small tossed salad
1 tbsp. salad dressing
1 cup skim milk
4 small oatmeal raisin cookies

Day 3: Tuesday

Breakfast

Maple Oats
½ bagel
1 tbsp. cream cheese
1 cup skim milk
½ cup orange juice

Lunch

Mexican restaurant/fast food
1 bean burrito
Tossed salad
1 tbsp. salad dressing

Afternoon Snack

1 cup fruit yogurt
3 tbsp. dry roasted peanuts

Dinner

Pasta con Cioppino
1 cup steamed zucchini and mushrooms sprinkled with Parmesan cheese
1 cup skim milk

Day 4: Wednesday

Breakfast

Fast 'n' Easy, Too
½ cup orange juice

Brown Bag Lunch

Turkey sandwich on hearty whole wheat
   bread with 1 oz. of turkey
Celery sticks
1 pear
2 Nature Valley Granola Bars (1 package)

Afternoon Snack

3 cups microwave popcorn

Dinner

Sesame Halibut
Tossed salad
2 tbsp. light salad dressing
1 corn on the cob
1 slice whole grain bread
2 tsp. butter or margarine
1 cup skim milk
½ cup frozen yogurt
4 small oatmeal raisin cookies

Day 5: Thursday

Breakfast

Sweet Sunshine
1 cup skim milk

Lunch

1 slice pizza with cheese
Tossed salad
2 tbsp. light salad dressing
1 slice garlic bread
1 cup skim milk

Afternoon Snack

1 apple
4 graham crackers
1 cup skim milk

Dinner

Easy Beans 'n' Rice
Tossed salad
2 tbsp. light salad dressing

Day 6: Friday
Breakfast
Old Reliable
½ cup orange juice

Brown Bag Lunch
Peanut butter and jelly sandwich on whole
   wheat
1 apple
Green and red pepper slices
1 cup skim milk

Afternoon snack
1 cup vanilla/coffee/lemon yogurt

Dinner
Enjoy a restaurant meal complete with dessert.

Day 7: Saturday
Breakfast
Breakfast Dessert
½ cinnamon-raisin bagel
1 tbsp. cream cheese

Lunch
Leftover Easy Beans 'n' Rice from Thursday
   night dinner
1 cup skim milk

Afternoon Snack
4 Fig Newtons
½ cup grapes

Dinner
Spaghetti Carbonara
Tossed salad
2 tbsp. salad dressing
½ cup frozen yogurt

Day 8: Sunday
Breakfast
2 pancakes
1 tbsp. maple syrup

1 cup skim milk
½ cup orange juice

Out for a Country Bike Tour or Picnic
Drink lots of water.

Packed Lunch on the Road
Peanut butter and apple butter on hearty
   whole wheat bread with 2 tbsp. peanut butter and 1 tbsp. apple butter
Carrot and celery sticks
1 apple
2 Nature Valley Granola Bars (1 package)

Packed Afternoon Snack
¼ cup dried apricots
4 graham cracker squares

Dinner
Enjoy a high-carbohydrate restaurant dinner.

Day 9: Monday
Breakfast
Breakfast Pizza
1 cup skim milk

Brown Bag Lunch
1 cup fruit yogurt
2 large squares Seasoned Ry-Krisp crackers
Handful of cherry tomatoes

Afternoon Snack
4 small oatmeal cookies

Dinner
Fried Tofu Pocket
Tossed salad
2 tbsp. light salad dressing
Fruit Smoothie

Day 10: Tuesday
Breakfast
Metro Special
1 cup skim milk

Lunch
Your best fast-food bet (see chapter 19 for a list)

Afternoon Snack
1 cup vanilla/coffee/lemon yogurt

Dinner
Sig's Slaw
1 corn on the cob
Small tossed salad
Fat-free salad dressing
1 cup skim milk

Day 11: Wednesday
Breakfast
Old Reliable
½ cup orange juice

Brown Bag Lunch
Leftover Sig's Slaw
1 pear

Afternoon Snack
4 Fig Newtons
1 cup skim milk

Dinner
Sesame Halibut
Tossed salad
2 tbsp. salad dressing
1 medium baked potato
1 slice whole grain bread
2 tsp. butter or margarine
1 cup skim milk

Day 12: Thursday
Breakfast
McBreakfast

Lunch
1 cup vanilla/coffee/lemon yogurt
1 apple

Afternoon Snack
1 oz. of pretzels
Your favorite flavor of sparkling water

Dinner
Curried Rice and Lentils
Tossed salad
2 tbsp. light salad dressing
1 cup skim milk

Day 13: Friday
Breakfast
Apples 'n' Cheese
1 cup skim milk

Brown Bag Lunch
Leftover Curried Rice and Lentils from last
    night's dinner
½ cup applesauce snack pack (1 package)

Afternoon Snack
2 tbsp. dry roasted peanuts
1 orange

Dinner
High-carbohydrate restaurant dinner

Day 14: Saturday
Breakfast
1 Aloha Muffin
1 cup skim milk

Lunch
1 cup bean soup
1 slice hearty whole wheat bread
Tossed salad
1 tbsp. salad dressing
1 apple
1 cup skim milk

Afternoon Snack

1 cup coffee/vanilla/lemon yogurt
½ large square Seasoned Ry-Krisp cracker

Dinner

Enjoy a restaurant dinner complete with
dessert.

Day 15: Sunday

Breakfast

½ cup orange juice
2 slices French toast
1 tbsp. maple syrup
1 cup skim milk
1 cup coffee

Out for a Hike

Drink lots of water.

Packed Lunch on the Road

Swiss cheese sandwich on hearty whole wheat
bread with 1 oz. of cheese
Carrot sticks
1 apple
2 Nature Valley Granola Bars (1 package)

Packed Afternoon Snack

¼ cup dried apricots
6 graham cracker squares

Dinner

Sesame Halibut
1 tossed salad
2 tbsp. salad dressing
1 small baked potato
1 tsp. butter or margarine
1 cup cooked broccoli (prepare 2 cups, with 1
cup for tomorrow's lunch)
1 square corn bread
1 cup frozen yogurt topped with fresh strawberries

Day 16: Monday

Breakfast

Maple Oats
½ grapefruit
1 cup skim milk

Lunch

1 cup fruit yogurt
2 squares corn bread from last night
1 cup cold cooked broccoli from last night with
1 tbsp. Italian dressing
1 pear

Afternoon Snack

2 Nature Valley Granola Bars (1 package)
1 cup skim milk

Dinner

Asparagus and Shrimp Stir-Fry
1 cup gingered rice
1 roll
2 tsp. butter
4 Fig Newtons

Day 17: Tuesday

Breakfast

Sweet Sunshine
1 cup skim milk

Lunch

Mexican restaurant/fast food
1 bean burrito
1 cup rice
Tossed salad
1 tbsp. salad dressing

Afternoon Snack

1 cup fruit yogurt
3 tbsp. dry roasted peanuts
1 cup vegetable juice

Dinner
Pasta con Cioppino
1 slice Italian garlic bread
1 cup steamed vegetables
1 cup skim milk

Day 18: Wednesday
Breakfast
Breakfast Dessert
½ bagel

Brown Bag Lunch
1 cup last night's leftover Pasta con Cioppino
heated in a microwave
Carrot and celery sticks
1 apple

Afternoon Snack
½ cup raisin and nut mixture

Dinner
Angelhair Scallops on a Spinach Bed
1 corn on the cob
1 roll
1 cup skim milk
½ cup frozen yogurt
2 graham cracker squares

Day 19: Thursday
Breakfast
Old Reliable
½ cup orange juice

Lunch
Your best fast-food bet (see chapter 19 for a list)

Afternoon Snack
1 cup vanilla/coffee/lemon yogurt
1 large square Seasoned Ry-Krisp cracker

Dinner
Sig's Slaw
1 hearty roll
1 corn on the cob
1 cup skim milk

Day 20: Friday
Breakfast
Fast 'n' Easy, Too

Brown Bag Lunch
Swiss cheese sandwich on hearty whole wheat
bread with 1 oz. of cheese
Carrot and celery sticks
1 pear

Afternoon Snack
2 Nature Valley Granola Bars (1 package)

Dinner
Easy Beans 'n' Rice
Large tossed salad
Fat-free salad dressing
1 cup skim milk
1 cup fresh berries with a dollop of vanilla yogurt

Day 21: Saturday
Breakfast
Metro Special
1 cup skim milk

Lunch
Large whole wheat pita stuffed with 1 oz.
cheese and lots of fresh veggies

Afternoon Snack
1 cup fruit yogurt

Dinner

Enjoy a restaurant dinner complete with
dessert.

Day 22: Sunday

Breakfast

2 pancakes
2 tbsp. maple syrup
1 cup skim milk
½ cup orange juice

Out for a Country Bike Tour

Drink lots of water.

Packed Lunch on the Road

Peanut butter and apple butter on hearty
whole wheat bread with 2 tbsp. peanut butter and 1 tbsp. apple butter
Carrot sticks
1 apple
2 Nature Valley Granola Bars (1 package)

Packed Afternoon Snack

¼ cup dried apricots
6 graham cracker squares

Dinner

Grilled Honey Yogurt Chicken (½ breast)
1 tossed salad
2 tbsp. fat-free salad dressing
1 cup pineapple rice
1 tsp. butter or margarine
1 cup cooked broccoli
1 slice crispy French bread
1 cup frozen yogurt

Day 23: Monday

Breakfast

Old Reliable

Brown Bag Lunch

Cold grilled chicken from last night's dinner
(½ breast)
Green pepper and cucumber slices
1 cup skim milk

Afternoon Snack

1 cup vanilla/coffee/ lemon yogurt
2 Fig Newtons

Dinner

Sig's Slaw
2 hearty rolls
1 corn on the cob
2 oatmeal raisin cookies

Day 24: Tuesday

Breakfast

Breakfast pizza

Lunch

Enjoy an ethnic vegetarian restaurant
delight.

Afternoon Snack

3 cups microwave popcorn
1 cup fruit juice
1 apple

Dinner

Sesame Halibut
Small tossed salad
1 tbsp. light salad dressing
1 medium baked sweet potato
1 slice whole grain bread
2 tsp. butter or margarine
1 cup skim milk
1 cup frozen yogurt
4 small oatmeal raisin cookies

Day 25: Wednesday

Breakfast

Maple Oats
1 cup skim milk

Brown Bag Lunch

1 cup fruit yogurt
2 large squares Seasoned Ry-Krisp crackers
Handful of cherry tomatoes and cucumber
   slices

Afternoon Snack

1 oz. pretzels
1 orange

Dinner

Fried Tofu Pocket
1 cup brown rice
Small tossed salad
2 tbsp. fat-free salad dressing
½ cup frozen yogurt

Day 26: Thursday

Breakfast

Old Reliable
½ cup orange juice

Lunch

Your best fast-food bet (see chapter 19 for a
   list)

Afternoon Snack

2 graham crackers
1 cup skim milk

Dinner

Easy Beans 'n' Rice
Tossed salad
2 tbsp. light salad dressing
½ cup sorbet with fresh raspberries

Day 27: Friday

Breakfast

Sweet Sunshine
1 cup skim milk

Brown Bag Lunch

1 cup vanilla/coffee/lemon yogurt
1 apple
Green and red pepper slices
1 cup skim milk

Afternoon Snack

½ cup grapes

Dinner

Enjoy a high-carbohydrate restaurant meal.

Day 28: Saturday

Breakfast

Breakfast Dessert
1 English muffin

Lunch

1 cup bean soup
2 slices hearty whole wheat bread
Tossed salad
1 tbsp. salad dressing
1 cup skim milk

Afternoon Snack

1 cup vanilla/coffee/lemon yogurt

Dinner

Enjoy a night on the town complete with
   dessert.

Day 29: Sunday

Breakfast

½ cup orange juice
2 slices French toast

1 cup skim milk
1 cup coffee

Out for a Hike

Drink lots of water.

Packed Lunch on the Road

Swiss cheese sandwich on hearty whole wheat
  bread with 1 oz. of cheese
Carrot and celery sticks
1 apple
2 Nature Valley Granola Bars (1 package)

Packed Afternoon Snack

¼ cup dried apricots
4 graham cracker squares

Dinner

Angelhair Scallops on a Spinach Bed
1 large baked sweet potato
1 large square corn bread
1 cup frozen yogurt topped with fresh strawberries

Day 30: Monday

Breakfast

Fast 'n' Easy, Too

Lunch

2 slices pizza with cheese
Small tossed salad
1 tbsp. salad dressing

Afternoon Snack

1 cup fruit yogurt
1 large square Seasoned Ry-Krisp cracker

Dinner

Curried Rice and Lentils
1 roll
Tossed salad
2 tbsp. light salad dressing
½ cup frozen yogurt with fresh berries

The High-Performance Nutrition Prescription Chart for Your Activity

Nutrients	Endurance-Type Exercisers	Strength Trainers	Cross Trainers
Major Nutrients			
Carbohydrates	60 to 65 percent of total calories	65 to 70 percent of total calories	60 to 70 percent of total calories
Protein	15 percent of total calories/.5 gram per pound of body weight daily	15 percent of total calories/.7 gram per pound of body weight daily	15 percent of total calories/.9 gram per pound of body weight daily
Fat	20 to 25 percent of total calories	20 to 25 percent of total calories	20 to 25 percent of total calories
Liquid Supplements			
Fluid-electrolyte	Before, during, or after workout	Before, during, or after workout	Before, during, or after workout
Carb supplement	After a workout; with or between meals	After a workout; with or between meals	After a workout; with or between meals
Meal replacer	With or between meals	8 oz. immediately following a workout	8 oz. immediately following a strength training workout; also use as a meal or snack
Creatine	Not indicated	2 g daily	2 g daily for short burst power sports
Antioxidants			
Vitamin C	200 to 300 mg daily	200 to 300 mg daily	200 to 300 mg daily
Vitamin E	100 to 400 IU daily	100 to 400 IU daily	100 to 400 IU daily

Nutrients	Endurance-Type Exercisers	Strength Trainers	Cross Trainers
Beta-carotene	10,000 to 20,000 IU daily	10,000 to 20,000 IU daily	10,000 to 20,000 IU daily
Selenium	Up to 50 μg daily	Up to 50 μg daily	Up to 50 μg daily
Sodium	Ultraendurance events lasting longer than 4 hours: drink a ½ to ¾ cup of a fluid-electrolyte drink every 10 to 20 minutes during the event	No supplementation indicated	No supplementation indicated unless cross training involves an ultraendurance event like a triathlon
Water			
Before exercise	8 to 16 oz. two hours prior to exercise; 4 to 8 oz. immediately before. In extremes of temperature: 12 to 20 oz. 10 to 20 minutes prior to exercise	8 to 16 oz. two hours prior to exercise; 4 to 8 oz. immediately before. In extremes of temperature: 12 to 20 oz. 10 to 20 minutes prior to exercise	8 to 16 oz. two hours prior to exercise; 4 to 8 oz. immediately before. In extremes of temperature: 12 to 20 oz. 10 to 20 minutes prior to exercise
During exercise	4 to 8 oz. every 15 to 20 minutes	4 to 8 oz. every 15 to 20 minutes	4 to 8 oz. every 15 to 20 minutes
After exercise	2 cups of water for every pound of lost body weight	2 cups of water for every pound of lost body weight	2 cups of water for every pound of lost body weight

APPENDIX C

On the Mend with High-Performance Nutrition

It happens to the best of us: an injury. It could be a backache, pulled muscle, torn ligament, skin injury, a fracture, a broken bone, or other exercise- or sports-related injury. Depending on the severity, you could be sidelined for a few weeks, a few months, even longer. If so, what adjustments do you make in your nutrition, if any? Here's a rundown.

Adequate Calories for Healing

Injured and out of commission, you're naturally going to need fewer calories. Keeping your calories at your active, preinjury level could lead to a weight gain, which would undo a lot of the good you've already done to your body.

So the first step is to reduce your daily caloric intake. If you're totally inactive during your recuperation, think of yourself as a sedentary person. To figure the number of calories you need, use the formula explained in chapter 17. Simply multiply your healthy weight by 10. Next, multiply your healthy weight by 3. Add the two numbers together to arrive at the calories you need to maintain your weight. So at a weight of 125, you would need 1,625 calories a day [(125 × 10 = 1,250) + (125 × 3 = 375) = 1,625].

Sixty-five percent of those calories should still come from complex carbohydrates, since these supply many of the nutrients your body needs for healing. Carbs like whole grains, fresh fruits, and vegetables will help prevent constipation caused by bed rest or inactivity.

Regardless of what your appetite may be, keep your calories at the recommended level for your body weight. Your body does need energy from calories to heal, especially if you have a broken bone. In that case, your diet must provide enough energy in the form of calories to manufacture new bone cells.

Protein Requirements

Since you're basically sedentary during your recuperation, you should drop your protein requirements to the recommended dietary allowance (RDA) for protein of .36 g per pound of body weight per day. Don't forgo protein, however, since it's so essential for rebuilding body tissue. When you're injured, your body immediately starts breaking down muscle protein to provide the energy required to repair damaged tissues. So without adequate protein in your diet, your rate of healing could slow down to less than what's considered its normal rate.

Nutritional Therapy

No single nutrient will make you heal faster. The best medicine is to follow your physician's orders, get the rest you need, and continue to eat properly. A healthy, balanced diet will supply the nutrients you need to repair body tissue and possibly counteract some of the stress caused by the injury. Make sure your diet during recuperation includes foods rich in the following nutrients:

Vitamin C. In the early stages of an injury, the body's stores of vitamin C are rapidly used up. Hopefully, if you were well nourished prior to the injury, you'll have a pool of vitamin C in your body to meet your immediate needs.

Vitamin C is necessary for the formation of collagen tissue for wound repair. With a deficiency of vitamin C, wound healing is likely to be slow. Your body doesn't store vitamin C, so you have to have a good source of this nutrient every day. Some healthy sources include citrus fruits, strawberries, tomatoes, and green peppers.

Zinc. This trace mineral is involved in the manufacture of protein used to repair damaged tissue. The requirement for zinc increases when the body is in a healing mode, although we don't know how much extra is actually needed. Don't start popping zinc supplements, either, since too much of this mineral can interfere with calcium absorption. Protein foods and whole grain products are usually high in zinc.

Calcium. If you've broken or fractured a bone, the immobilization that the injury causes can lead to calcium losses. Plus, if you're not getting enough calcium during your recuperation, your body will tap into your healthy bones to get the calcium it needs to fix your broken bone. All this spells trouble. You absolutely must get your RDA of calcium while recuperating, and a little more wouldn't hurt. Food sources of calcium include milk, low-fat dairy products, and some vegetables.

Antioxidants.   In addition to the nutrients you're getting from your meals, continue to take an antioxidant supplement once a day. Antioxidants have a role to play in helping tissues mend and regenerate.

Clearly, a healthful diet will help keep you on the mend, and it's best to get the nutritional resources you need from food. Of course, nutritional therapy is just one part of getting better and only an adjunct, never a substitute, for your physician's treatment plan.

Medication and Nutrition Guide

As an exerciser or athlete, you're eating healthy portions of food and perhaps taking supplements. Occasionally, you may have to take medication, like an anti-inflammatory drugs for joint pain or a pulled muscle, or antibiotics for an infection. What many people don't realize is that some medications can interfere with good nutrition, unless you know how to take them properly and at what times.

Certain foods and drugs taken in combination can often cancel out each other's benefits. As discussed earlier, food is a combination of thousands of chemicals. Drugs are also chemicals. When mixed together, these chemicals can interact with one another, changing the way they work inside your body. For example, minerals from foods or supplements may bind with drugs in the intestines and reduce the total amount of the drug absorbed. If less than the recommended dosage is absorbed, the drug may not work as well. Drugs may also make your body lose minerals. This potentially compromises your nutritional health, especially if you take the medication in question for a long time.

Not all drugs interact with foods, however. But many are influenced by when and what we eat. Food can delay or cut the absorption of many drugs. The effect of the drug isn't changed, but the time it takes to act is prolonged. That's why you're often told to take certain medications on an empty stomach. Some drugs can irritate the stomach, though, and should be taken with food.

To help you get the most from your nutrition and medication, here's a guide to the drugs used most frequently by active people, with information on planning your meals around them.

Nonsteroidal Anti-inflammatory Drugs (NSAIDs)

Commonly taken for inflammation and pain, these drugs are available both over-the-counter and by prescription. Ibuprofen is the most widely available over-the-counter NSAID, and brand names include Advil, Motrin, Nuprin, and Rufen. A newer medication is naproxen, sold as Aleve.

NSAIDs should be taken with food, since they may irritate the stomach lining. Other side effects that may affect nutritional health include nausea, bloating, gas, constipation, vomiting, loss of appetite, and diarrhea. Avoid drinking alcohol with these drugs.

Antibiotics

For better absorption, always take antibiotics with a glass of water on an empty stomach, unless otherwise noted by a physician or pharmacist. In susceptible people, antibiotics can cause stomach and intestinal upset, including nausea, vomiting, and diarrhea.

Because of these side effects, many people mistakenly believe they should take antibiotics with milk (rather than water) to "coat their stomachs." But if some antibiotics—notably tetracycline—are taken with milk, the calcium, magnesium, iron, and zinc in the milk will bind with the drug, interfering with its absorption and action in the body.

Asthma Preparations

Beta-agonist inhalers, which many active people take for asthma, have no known interactions with food. Theophylline is a bronchodilator commonly prescribed for asthma. Brand medications include Bronkodyl, Theobid, Theodur, Theolair, and Theo-24. Take these medications on an empty stomach and avoid a diet excessively high in protein or carbohydrate. Carbohydrate loading, for instance, would not be recommended during theophylline treatment. Theophylline is a chemical cousin of caffeine, so caffeine-containing foods should be limited while taking this drug. So should charcoal-broiled foods.

Side effects of theophylline that may hurt your nutritional health include nausea, vomiting (may include vomiting of blood), stomach upset, diarrhea, increased thirst, anorexia, and hyperglycemia (an excess of sugar in the blood).

Tedral is a theophylline preparation that also includes other drug compounds, ephedrine and phenobarbital. For better absorption, take Tedral with a glass of water on an empty stomach.

Antihypertensive Medications

Some of the diuretics prescribed for the treatment of high blood pressure can promote mineral loss. Furosemide (Lasix) and hydrochlorothiazide (HydroDIURIL) increase potassium and magnesium losses. If you take these medications long term, add foods to your diet that are high in potassium (bananas, oranges, potatoes) and magnesium (nuts, legumes, whole grains) to avoid depleting your body of these minerals. A low-sodium diet is commonly prescribed with antihypertensive medications. Therefore, you shouldn't eat natural licorice, which tends to enhance sodium retention.

Take diuretics with food at least three hours before bedtime. Avoid foods containing sorbitol (found in many dietetic and sugar-free foods) because they may cause diarrhea and result in excessive fluid loss. To avoid dehydration, limit your alcohol consumption to 1 to 2 oz. occasionally and only with the advice of your physician. Other nutritionally related side effects include nausea, vomiting, anorexia, dry mouth, increased thirst, and possibly a peculiar sweet taste in the mouth.

Beta-blockers, another type of antihypertensive medication, should be taken with food at the same time each day. Propranolol HCl (Inderal) is the most commonly prescribed beta-blocker.

Antacids

Antacids, such as Maalox and Mylanta, are composed of aluminum and magnesium hydroxides. These may cut the absorption of vitamin A. If you continually use these antacids, you may end up with diminished absorption of calcium. And overuse of them may lead to hypermagnesemia, or magnesium toxicity. Take antacids one hour after meals or between meals.

The antacid Tums is formulated from calcium carbonate, of which 40 percent is used as calcium by the body. If you take Tums for an upset stomach, don't ingest large amounts of dairy products at the same time because the protein in these foods will increase acid secretions. As a calcium supplement, Tums should not be taken with high-fiber foods or foods high in oxalates (greens, tea), since these compounds will bind the mineral and interfere with absorption.

Laxatives

As a general rule, you should be on a high-fiber diet so that you don't need laxatives. Frequent and prolonged use of any laxative can flush electrolytes, particularly potassium, from your body. Take laxatives on an empty stomach with a glass of water. Don't take them within one hour of eating or drinking dairy products because they can bind with the calcium and decrease absorption.

Antiviral Medications

The antiviral acyclovir (Zovirax) is taken to treat initial episodes of the herpes virus and help prevent its recurrence. You can take it with food, but be sure to also

Table D-1

GENERAL GUIDELINES FOR TAKING MEDICATIONS*

- Always read your prescription label. If you don't understand something, or feel that you need more information, ask your physician or pharmacist.
- Read all directions, warnings, and interaction precautions printed on labels and packages. Don't assume that taking over-the-counter medications is problem-free.
- Take medications with a full glass of water to enhance absorption and utilization.
- Never take medications with alcohol.
- Don't mix medications with hot drinks. This may destroy the effectiveness of the drug.
- Don't mix medications with food, unless instructed to do so. This may alter the drug's effectiveness.
- Because nutrients can alter the effect of drugs, don't take vitamin-mineral supplements with medications.

*Source: "Food and Drugs. When Don't They Mix?" *Mayo Clinic Health Letter* (April 1991), p. 4.

drink about eight glasses of fluids during treatment (especially if you're physically active) to make sure the medicine clears from your body.

Table D-1 provides a summary of the guidelines to use when taking medications.

Your Personal Diet and Training Logs

Keeping daily logs of your diet and exercise activities is a great way to stay on the straight and narrow. If you're trying to lose weight, for example, a daily record can pinpoint red flags that are contributing to overeating and body fat gain.

Following the discussion here, you'll find sample templates for diet, training (for exercise, rest, and work), and supplements and medication. I use these same forms in my practice with great success. They're a great motivational tool. You'll be able to learn something from each piece of information you record, as described next.

Body weight: Changes in your weight provide a wealth of information, including how close you are to attaining your fitness goals. Also, a sudden drop or elevation in weight could signal a serious medical problem. Record your body weight only once a week. Daily fluctuations are insignificant. Try to weigh yourself on the same scale, at the same time of day, with similar clothing. But remember, your body weight may not reflect healthy changes in body composition or body measurements.

Type of food, description, and amount: You may find out that you're eating too much of something or that it's prepared with a lot of fat.

Location: Where you eat can be a real eye-opener, too. Restaurants or parties, for example, may be places where you tend to indulge in high-fat, high-sugar foods.

Your feelings: Emotions can cause us to slip into bad eating habits. Sometimes we overeat when we're depressed—or happy. Other times, we may undereat or not eat at all. Hunger is a telltale sign, too. Eating when you're not hungry, for example, could lead to excessive caloric intake. Or maybe you feel hungry most of the time. In that case, you may not be eating enough calories to fuel your energy needs.

Exercise: How much are you doing—and for how long? What type of exercise are you performing? Over time, you may detect some patterns. For example, the more aerobics you do, the leaner you get. But maybe you're not as toned or as strong as you'd like to be. An increase in the amount of strength training you're doing might be in order.

Also, recording your sets and reps in strength training is critical. To make progress, you must keep trying to perform more work, either heavier weights, more reps, and a combination of the two. By challenging your muscles in this manner, you'll make greater gains. The best way to chart your progress is by writing it down.

Energy level: Some days you may feel full of energy; other times, as if you're dragging. Comparing your diet log with your training log may reveal that certain foods give you greater energy to perform. If so, you may want to fine-tune your diet and add more energy-giving foods.

Supplements/medications: Recording this information helps you keep track of what you're taking.

Amount/dose/frequency: This information helps you avoid dangerous megadosing (supplements) or overdosing (medications), as well as supplement/drug interactions.

DIET LOG

Day:		Date:		Body Weight:	
Today's Diet:					
Time of Day	**Food Eaten**	**Description**	**Quantity**	**Location**	**How you felt, why you ate**
Example:					
12 noon	Chicken breast Broccoli	Broiled, no skin Steamed	Half 4 stalks	Home	Hungry

TRAINING LOG

Day:	Date:	Body Weight:
Today I feel:		
Today's Training:		

Time	Exercise	Reps and Sets/Time/Distance

SUPPLEMENTATION/MEDICATION LOG

Day:	Date:	Body Weight:
Today's Nutritional Supplements and Medications:		
Supplement/Medications	**Amount/Dose**	**Frequency**
Example:		
Vitamin C Oat bran Ibuprofen	250 mg 3 tbsp. 400 mg	1 time/day 1 time/day 3 times/day

Food Additives: A Guide for Physically Active People

Physically active people eat a lot of food, and in much of that food come additives, which can be harmful to health. I always caution exercisers and athletes about this, since they're at risk of consuming more additives than the average person.

Today about 2,800 additives are put into our foods. Additives keep food from spoiling; improve its appearance, texture, or taste; or fortify its nutritive value. The most frequently used additives are sugar, salt, and corn syrup. Others include nutrients, food coloring, flavor enhancers, preservatives, and synthetic chemicals.

Some additives unintentionally sneak into foods during growing, processing, packaging, or storing. Farmers, for example, spray their crops with pesticides to protect them from insect damage. Stored cereal grains and other farm commodities are often treated with pesticides to kill insects and reduce waste. Traces of pesticides can wind up in food.

Then there's the issue of treating livestock with drugs to keep them healthy. These drugs can end up contaminating our food supply. Under normal circumstances, infected dairy cows treated with antibiotics secrete the drugs in their milk. Batches of this milk are thrown out until only pure, untainted milk is produced. This practice is legal and usually safe. But if the drugs remain in the cow's body or the government fails to test the milk properly, you could drink contaminated milk. The same thing can happen with the meat of drug-treated animals or fish.

Other uses of additives are intentional. Food manufacturers use chemicals to enhance or stabilize the nutrients in foods, prevent bacterial contamination and spoilage, make food preparation more convenient, and expand the variety of foods available in the grocery store. Additives also increase a food's shelf life.

With the thousands of compounds being added to foods, is the stuff we eat becoming a chemical cocktail? Is all the variety and convenience worth it? More important, what are the risks to our health? Let's take a closer look at exactly what goes into our foods—and what it's doing to our bodies.

Are Food Colorings Unsafe?

Do bright fruits, fresh-looking luncheon meats, rich cheeses, and other tastefully displayed foods along the grocery store aisles make your mouth water?

If so, what's taunting your taste buds might not be the food but rather its color. There are thirty-three color additives approved by the FDA for use in foods. Some are natural, others are synthetic. A common natural coloring agent is beta-carotene, a nutrient that adds an orange, yellow, or red hue to products like margarine, cheese, and macaroni.

Synthetic coloring agents include seven compounds derived from coal tar, a by-product of coal: FD&C Blue No. 1, FD&C Green No. 3, FD&C Red No. 3, FD&C Red No. 40, and FD&C Yellow No. 5, Orange B, and Citrus Red No. 2. All but two are approved for general use in food. Orange B is limited to casings or surfaces of frankfurters and sausages, and Citrus Red No. 2 is used only in the skins of oranges.

About two out of every ten thousand people are allergic to FD&C Yellow No. 5 (also known as tartrazine), according to research. The symptoms include hives, itching, and nasal congestion. If you're allergic to aspirin, you may also be allergic to FD&C Yellow No. 5.

By law, foods containing this color must say so on the label. FD&C Yellow No. 5 is typically found in orange drinks, gelatin, cake mixes, processed cheese dinners, and snacks. Other approved colors aren't required to be listed by name but may be labeled as an artificial color, artificial coloring, or "color added."

MSG

Nearly two thousand flavoring agents are put into foods! Among the best known is monosodium glutamate, or MSG. It is a flavor enhancer found in seasonings such as the product Accent, and is frequently used to season Chinese cuisine.

As a kid, I occasionally ate at Chinese restaurants with my family. After a meal, I'd always get a temple-squeezing headache—a reaction I blamed on the tea served in the restaurant. Years later, it was revealed that eating MSG can trigger a nasty reaction in sensitive people. That was precisely my problem—a sensitivity to MSG.

Commonly known as the Chinese restaurant syndrome, this reaction affects one out of several hundred people, usually about twenty minutes after eating the additive. Frequently reported symptoms are burning sensations, chest and facial flushing or pain, and throbbing headaches. Although judged safe for use by adults, MSG should be avoided by infants, pregnant women, and others who are sensitive to it.

You can request that your food—with the exception of soup—be served without MSG. Even so, a lot of commercially prepared soups contain MSG, so be careful if you're sensitive like I am. I always make my own soups.

Nitrites and Other Bacteria-Fighting Agents

These preservatives halt the growth of bacteria responsible for food-borne diseases. Historically, sugar and salt are the most-often used bacteria-fighting agents. Others are potassium sorbate and sodium propionate, which also extend the shelf life of foods. Both are used extensively in baked goods, cheese, beverages, mayonnaise, margarine, and other products.

Among the most controversial bacteria-fighting agents are nitrites, a type of salt added to foods. Nitrites preserve the pink color of certain foods, particularly hot dogs and other cured meats, keep foods from turning rancid, and protect against botulinum, bacteria that produce a deadly toxin or poison when they grow in food.

The use of nitrites in foods is being closely studied. In the body, nitrites can be converted to compounds called *nitrosamines*. These are formed during digestion when nitric oxide and proteins called *amines* bond together. At nitrite levels higher than those used in foods, nitrosamine formation causes cancer in animals. It's not yet clear whether nitrosamines are carcinogenic in humans.

Antioxidants as Food Protectors

As food is exposed to air it changes chemically in a process known as *oxidation*. Oxidation causes food to spoil and turn rancid. Antioxidants are added to food to prevent these reactions. Twenty-seven antioxidants are approved as preservatives by the FDA, including vitamin C (ascorbate) and vitamin E (tocopherol).

Sulfites, sulfur-containing salts, are also considered antioxidants because they keep oxidation in check in many processed foods, dried fruits, alcoholic beverages, and drugs. Sulfites are not without their controversy, however. At one time, they were used on salad bars to keep raw fruits and vegetables looking fresh. This practice was banned in 1986 after documented cases revealed that 5 to 10 percent of people with asthma suffered severe reactions to sulfites. Some even died. Sulfites are now prohibited on all raw foods except grapes. Any food containing sulfites must list the additive on its label. Sulfites also destroy a significant amount of the B-complex vitamin thiamin in foods.

Two widely used antioxidants are the synthetic additives BHT and BHA, found as preservatives in cookies, crackers, and other baked foods. A newly discovered property of BHT and BHA is their ability to boost levels of a natural cancer fighter in laboratory animals and possibly in humans. In 1994 researchers at Cornell Medical College discovered that these preservatives activate the gene for an enzyme that helps defuse carcinogens before they can trigger tumor growth. Still, BHT and BHA are synthetic chemicals. I wouldn't put too much stock in this finding just yet.

Fortifying Food with Nutrients

Many refined and processed products are fortified by the addition of vitamins and minerals. Since the 1940s fortification of food has been a standard practice to alleviate certain nutritional deficiency disorders that were once prevalent in the United States. Grain products are enriched with iron, thiamin, riboflavin, and niacin. Iodine is added to salt, and vitamins A and D are put into dairy products.

Generally Recognized as Safe: But Are You the Exception?

What are additives doing to our bodies? Many of the answers remain to be seen. The FDA can only ensure that statistical risks to our health remain very small. Although the agency suggests a safety range for the consumption of additives and food substitutes, it can't safeguard you from unusual reactions, particularly if you don't follow the recommended guidelines.

A minimum number of studies is required to establish the safety of new products prior to FDA approval. After that, the products are listed as "generally recognized as safe" (GRAS). The population at large then becomes the laboratory. Most of us fall within the statistical average and will be able to use these products without risk to our health. Others will undoubtedly fall outside that norm, but there's no way to tell who the exceptions are. Eating these compounds one at a time might give you a clue as to whether you're sensitive to it. But this isn't too practical.

There's greater regulation of food additives now than at any other time in history. Even so, the FDA has taken the position that it can't provide absolute protection from all carcinogens. Instead, the agency now labels additives safe if they present no more than a one-in-a-million risk of cancer to human beings from a lifetime of use.

Food Irradiation

An alternative to chemical additives that is being considered is a preservative process called *food irradiation*. It treats food with radiation to kill pests and bacteria. In this process, food is conveyed through a lead-lined chamber where it's exposed to cobalt-60, a radioisotope that has been used in hospital settings for more than thirty years. FDA regulated, doses are carefully measured and monitored. The food has no chance to become contaminated with radioactivity.

Even so, this process raises some legitimate concerns. Studies have shown that food irradiation alters nutrients and chemicals in foods in much the same way canning, freezing, pasteurization, and cooking do. Not only that, irradiation forms new substances in foods not present prior to processing. As yet, we have no information on the health effects of consuming these by-products of irradiation.

Tests on the process are ongoing. However, the FDA has already given a preliminary go-ahead to irradiation within specified doses to spices, some meats, fruits, and vegetables. The process is supposed to thwart insect infestation, kill *Trichinella spiralis* (the pork parasite responsible for widespread disease), and keep tuberous vegetables like potatoes from sprouting.

But the jury is still out on whether irradiated foods are good for us. For a verdict, we need more data on the safety of irradiation versus chemical additives. At this time, all foods are required to be labeled if they undergo irradiation; however, a prepared food using an ingredient that has been irradiated need not state so on the label.

As consumers, it's our responsibility to be informed, to make wise choices, and to speak out when we feel strongly about an issue. Contact your local or regional FDA office to find out the status of food irradiation regulation, and you can submit your written opinions to the committee that makes the final decisions.

You can locate your local FDA office in the government pages of the phone book under U.S. Government, General Services Administration, Department of Health and Human Services, Food and Drug Administration.

Cutting Back on Additives

Additives and food substitutes still aren't the real thing, and health hazards are associated with them. Fortunately, you have considerable choice about what you eat. If you have a history of food allergies, read labels and avoid or limit foods that contain ingredients to which you are sensitive. If you have a reaction and think it may be related to a food additive, you or your doctor should contact the FDA.

There are ways you can cut back on the amount of food additives you eat, as well as keep your food from becoming contaminated with disease-causing germs. Some suggestions:

✔ Buy food fresh and store it properly. Observe "use by" or "sell by" dates on cartons. Buy fresh fish that has been kept frozen or on ice. Keep food properly refrigerated, not leaving it out for longer than two hours. Thaw food in the refrigerator or microwave and use immediately.

✔ Handle and prepare food safely. Wash all fruits and vegetables thoroughly. Remove outer leaves and peel when appropriate. Cook eggs, meat, fish, and poultry thoroughly to kill harmful bacteria that may be present. Use a meat thermometer, and cook meat to the following internal temperatures:

beef: 160°F   veal: 170°F
lamb: 170°F   pork: 170°F
poultry: 180–185°F   stuffing: 165°F
boneless turkey roast: 170–175°F

After handling raw eggs, meat, fish, and poultry, wash hands and all utensils in soapy water to avoid "cross-contamination" to the cooked product or other foods.

✔ Try to obtain *certified organic products* whenever possible. There is no federally regulated definition for the term *organic,* but twenty-one states have instituted organic programs or statute definitions. Recently, the federal government did pass a law addressing terms for organic farming regulation, but there has been a delay in instituting the law. Plans are under way to get it going soon. Your local or state USDA office can help you find out more information.

The term *organic* doesn't describe how nutritious a food is. Instead, according to the California definition, it means that the food has been produced, stored, processed, and packaged without the use of synthetic fertilizers, herbicides, fungicides, or pesticides, for one year prior to the appearance of flower buds in the case of perennial crops, and one year prior to seed planting in the case of annual crops. Other states require more years to establish certified organic farms.

In states without legal organic regulations, many cooperative growing communities have established their own standards. Others work with the Organic Crop Improvement Association (OCIA), an independent inspection and certification body. The OCIA seal of certification is recognized worldwide.

Even with these regulations, runoff water, soil shifting, and pesticides floating in the air may still cause chemicals to collect on foods. Therefore, it's important to always clean and wash fresh fruits and vegetables thoroughly.

✔ Choose safe food. Because most chemicals are fat soluble, they are stored in the fat of animals. Choose the leanest meat and fish products, and then remove the visible sources of fat before cooking. Select fish caught in cleaner waters far off shore, such as cod, haddock, and pollock. Even though salmon is found closer to shore, it's also a good selection.

✔ Limit your intake of packaged and highly processed convenience foods. These are chemical and preservative-laden. So are processed meats like cold cuts. Use fresh meat or poultry products instead. Read ingredient lists on food labels and avoid products containing questionable additives.

✔ Demand a safer marketplace. Speak out and let government officials know that you're not satisfied with the level of safety in our food supply. As hard as we may try, we can do very little on our own about some food safety problems, but if all of us speak out, we can make a difference.

REFERENCES

Chapter 1: Eating for Performance and Health

Butler, R. N. "Did You Say 'Sarcopenia'? (Muscle Mass Reduction)." *Geriatrics* 648, no. 2 (1993): 11–12.

Pasmantier, R. M. "Work Out Your Body and Mind to Slow Down the Aging Process." *Diabetes in the News* 12, no. 5 (1993): 6–8.

Rogers, M. A., and W. J. Evans. "Changes in Skeletal Muscle with Aging: Effects of Exercise Training." *Exercise in Sports Sciences Review* 21 (1993): 65–66.

Shepard, R. J. "Exercise and Aging: Extending Independence in Older Adults." *Geriatrics* 48, no. 5 (1993): 61–64.

Chapter 2: Carbohydrates

Rosencrans, J. "High-Fiber Vegetables, Fruits, Grains Are Pasta Alternative." *The Evansville* (Ind.) *Courier,* 22 February 1995, B2.

Chapter 3: Carbohydrates for Exercise and Competition

Walberg-Rankin, J. "Ergogenic Effects of Carbohydrate Intake during Long- and Short-Term Exercise." Paper presented at Nutritional Ergogenic Aids Conference sponsored by the Gatorade Sports Institute, November 11–12, 1994, Chicago.

Chapter 4: Fat

Muoio, D., J. J. Leddy, P. J. Horvath, et al. "Effect of Dietary Fat on Metabolic Adjustments to Maximal VO_2 and Endurance in Runners." *Medicine and Science in Sports and Exercise* 26, no. 1 (1994): 81–88.

Chapter 5: Protein

Davis, J. M. "Carbohydrates, Branched Chain Amino Acids and Endurance: The Central Fatigue Hypothesis." Paper presented at Nutritional Ergogenic Aids Conference sponsored by the Gatorade Sports Institute, November 11–12, 1994, Chicago.

Lemon, P. "Dietary Protein and Amino Acids." Paper presented at Nutritional Ergogenic Aids Conference sponsored by the Gatorade Sports Institute, November 11–12, 1994, Chicago.

Scripps Howard News Service. "Kidney Cancer Linked to Protein." *The Evansville* (Ind.) *Courier,* 16 August 1994.

Chapter 6: Phytochemicals

American Institute for Cancer Research Newsletter 46 (winter 1995): 11.

Begley, S. "Beyond Vitamins." *Newsweek,* 25 April 1994, 44–49.

Cassidy, A., S. Bingham, and K. D. R. Setchell. "Biological Effects of a Diet of Soy Protein Rich in Isoflavones on the Menstrual Cycle of Premenopausal Women." *American Journal of Clinical Nutrition* 60 (1994): 333–40.

Dwyer, J.T., B. R. Goldin, N. Sual, et al. "Tofu and Soy Drinks Contain Phytoestrogens." *Journal of the American Dietetic Association* 94, no. 7 (1994): 739–43.

Liebman, B. "Designer Foods." *Nutrition Action Newsletter* 18, no. 3 (1991): 1–4.

Messina, M. J. "Dietary Phytoestrogens: Cancer Cause or Prevention." *The Soy Connection* 3, no. 1 (1994): 1–4.

Messina, M.J., and V. Messina. *The Simple Soybean and Your Health,* p. 72. New York: Avery Publishing Group, 1994.

Zava, D. T. "The Phytoestrogen Paradox." *The Soy Connection* 3, no. 1 (1994): 1–4.

Chapter 7: Vitamins

"Antioxidants and the Elite Athlete." Published proceedings of the panel discussion at the 39th Annual Meeting of the American College of Sports Medicine, May 27, 1992, Dallas.

Higgins, L. C. "Longevity: An Eternal Quest Quickens." *Medical World News* 31, no. 10 (1990): 22–26.

Kanter, M. M. "Antioxidants and Other Popular Ergogenic Aids." From the proceedings of the Nutritional Ergogenic Aids Conference, November 11–12, 1994, Chicago.

National Research Council. *Diet and Health—Implications for Reducing Chronic Disease Risk,* p. 331. Washington, DC: National Academy Press, 1989.

O'Shea, M. "Better Fitness." *Parade Magazine,* December 18, 1994, p. 19.

Stampfer, M. J., C. H. Hennekens, J. E. Manson, G.A. Colditz, B. Rosner, and W. C. Willett. "Vitamin E Consumption and the Risk of Coronary Disease in Women." *New England Journal of Medicine* 328 (1993): 1444–49.

Rimm, E. B., M. J. Stampfer, A. Ascherio, E. Giovannucci, G. A. Colditz , and W. C. Willett. "Vitamin E Consumption and the Risk of Coronary Heart Disease in Men." *New England Journal of Medicine* 328 (1993): 1450–56.

Toufexis, A. "The New Scoop on Vitamins." *Time,* 6 April 1992, 54–59.

Chapter 8: Minerals

Bales, C. "Nutritional Aspects of Osteoporosis. Recommendations for the Elderly at Risk." *Annual Review of Gerontology and Geriatrics* 9 (1989): 7–34.

Consensus Conference on Osteoporosis. "Statement." *Journal of the American Medical Association* 252 (1984): 299–802.

Jenkins, R. R. "Exercise, Oxidative Stress, and Antioxidants: A Review." *International Journal of Sport Nutrition* 3 (1993): 356–75.

Lukaski, H. "Micronutrients: Are Mineral Supplements Necessary in the Athlete's Diet?" Paper presented at the Nutritional Ergogenic Aids Conference sponsored by the Gatorade Sports Institute, November 11–12, 1994, Chicago.

National Research Council. *Diet and Health—Implications for Reducing Chronic Disease Risk.* Washington, DC: National Academy Press,1989.

Chapter 9: Antioxidant Supplementation

"Antioxidants and the Elite Athlete." Published proceedings of the panel discussion at the 39th Annual Meeting of the American College of Sports Medicine, May 27, 1992, Dallas.

Daily, P. O., and P. T. Milligan. "Antioxidants: Clearing the Confusion." *Idea Today,* September 1994, 67–73.

Kanter, M. M., L. A. Nolte, and J. O. Holloszy. "Effects of an Antioxidant Vitamin Mixture on Lipid Peroxidation at Rest and Postexercise." *Journal of Applied Physiology* 74, no. 2 (1993): 965–69.

Meydani, M., W. J. Evans, G. Handelman, et al. "Protective Effect of Vitamin E on Exercise-Induced Oxidative Damage in Young and Older Adults." *American Journal of Physiology* 264, no. 5, Pt. 2 (1993): R992–98.

Chapter 10: Creatine: The Antidote to Low Energy

"Creatine Propels British Athletes to Olympic Gold Medals: Is Creatine the One True Ergogenic Aid?" *Running Research News* 9, no. 1 (1993): 1–5.

Greenhaff, P. "Can Creatine Loading Improve High Power Performance?" Paper presented at the Nutritional Ergogenic Aids Conference sponsored by the Gatorade Sports Institute, November 11–12, 1994, Chicago.

Hirvonen, J., A. Numela, H. Rusko, et al. "Fatigue and Changes of ATP, Creatine Phosphate, and Lactate during the 400-m Sprint." *Canadian Journal of Sports Science* 17 (1992): 141–44. Reported by B. Leibovitz. "Creatine: Energy-Storing Molecule in Muscle and Ergogenic Aid." *Muscular Development* 30, no. 11 (1993): 74, 156.

"The Promise of Creatine Supplements." *Penn State Sports Medicine Newsletter* 2, no. 5 (1994): 1–3.

Chapter 11: My Firming Formula

Chandler, R. M., H. K. Byrne, J. G. Patterson, and J. L. Ivy. "Dietary Supplements Affect the Anabolic Hormones After Weight-Training Exercise." *Journal of Applied Physiology* 76, no. 2 (1994): 839–45.

Fahey, T. D., K. Hoffman, W. Colvin, and G. Lauten. "The Effects of Intermittent Liquid Meal Feeding on Selected Hormones and Substrates during Intense Weight Training." *International Journal of Sport Nutrition* 3 (1993): 67–75.

Keim, N. L., B. L. Anderson, T. F. Barbieri, and M. Wu. "Moderate Diet Restriction Alters the Substrate and Hormone Response to Exercise." *Medicine and Science in Sports and Exercise* 26, no. 5 (1994): 599–604.

Maresh, C. M., L. E. Armstrong, J. R. Hoffman, D. R. Hannon, et al. "Dietary Supplementation and Improved Anaerobic Performance." *International Journal of Sport Nutrition* 4 (1994): 387–397.

Spiller, G.A., C. D. Jensen, T. S. Pattison, C. S. Chuck, et al. "Effect of Protein Dose on Serum Glucose and Insulin Response to Sugars." *American Journal of Clinical Nutrition* 46, no. 3 (1987): 474–80.

Zawadzki, K. M., B. B. Yaselkis, and J. L. Ivy. "Carbohydrate-Protein Complex Increases the Rate of Muscle Glycogen Storage after Exercise." *Journal of Applied Physiology* 75, no. 5 (1992): 1854–59.

Chapter 12: The Truth about Some Supplements

Brass, E. P., C. L. Hoppel, and W. R. Hiatt, "Effect of Intravenous L-Carnitine on Carnitine Homeostasis and Fuel Metabolism during Exercise in Humans." *Clinical Pharmacology and Therapeutics* 55, no. 6 (1994): 681–92.

Clancy, S. P., P. M. Clarkson, M. E. DeCheke, et al. "Effects of Chromium Picolinate Supplementation on Body Composition, Strength, and Urinary Chromium Loss in Football Players." *International Journal of Sport Nutrition* 4 (1994):142–53.

Clarkson, P. M. "Nutritional Ergogenic Aids: Carnitine." *International Journal of Sport Nutrition* 2 (1992):185–90.

Cowart, V. S. "Dietary Supplements: Alternatives to Anabolic Steroids?" *The Physician and Sportsmedicine* 20, no. 3 (1992): 189–98.

"Diet Supplement May Be Tainted." *Evansville* (Ind.) *Courier,* 31 August 1994, A7.

Jacobsen, B. H. "Effect of Amino Acids on Growth Hormone Release." *The Physician and Sportsmedicine* 18, no. 1 (1990): 68.

Kanter, M. M. "Antioxidants and Other Popular Ergogenic Aids." From the proceedings of the Nutritional Ergogenic Aids Conference, November 11–12, 1994, Chicago.

Kanter, M. M. "Free Radicals, Exercise, and Antioxidant Supplementation." *International Journal of Sport Nutrition* 4 (1994): 205–20.

Lambert, M. I., et al. "Failure of Commercial Oral Amino Acid Supplements to Increase Serum Growth Hormone Concentrations in Male Body-Builders." *International Journal of Sport Nutrition* 3 (1993): 298–305.

Lefavi, R. G., R. A. Anderson, R. E. Keith, et al. "Efficacy of Chromium Supplementation in Athletes: Emphasis on Anabolism." *International Journal of Sport Nutrition* 2 (1992): 111–22.

Lukaski, H. "Micronutrients: Are Mineral Supplements Necessary in the Athlete's Diet?" From the proceedings of the Nutritional Ergogenic Aids Conference, November 11–12, 1994, Chicago.

Nielsen, F. H. "Boron—An Overlooked Element of Potential Nutritional Importance." *Nutrition Today* 23, no. 1 (1988): 4–7.

Chapter 13: Herbal Supplements

Breum, L., J. K. Pedersen, F. Ahlstrom, et al. "Comparison of an Ephedrine/Caffeine Combination and Dexfenfluramine in the Treatment of Obesity—A Double-Blind Multi-Centre Trial in General Practice." *International Journal of Obesity Related Metabolic Disorders* 18, no. 2 (1994): 99–103.

Catlin, D. H., M. Sekera, and D. C. Adelman, "Erthroderma Associated with Ingestion of an Herbal Product." *The Western Journal of Medicine* 159, no. 4 (1993): 491–94.

Hendler, S. S. "Tapping the Healing Power of Herbs." *Executive Health's Good Health Report* 28, no. 8 (1992): 1–4.

"Herbs, Like Drugs, Have a Dark Side." *Environmental Nutrition* 16, no. 11 (1993): 8.

Hobbs, C. "Adaptogens: All-Purpose Herbs." *East West* 21, no. 7 (1991): 54–61.

McCaleb, R. "Ginseng Energy Booster: This Popular Ancient Herb Is Used to Boost Immunity and Energy and to Increase Strength." *Better Nutrition for Today's Living* 54, no. 1 (1992): 34–36.

The Milwaukee Journal-Scripps Howard News Service. "DEA Fears Potent New Drug Spread: Highly Addictive and Easily Produced Stimulant Shows Up." *The Evansville* (Ind.) *Courier,* 24 June 1993, C4.

Pieralisi, G., P. Ripari, and L. Vecchiet. "Effects of a Standardized Ginseng Extract Combined with Dimethylaminoethanol Bitartrate, Vitamins, Minerals, and Trace Elements on Physical Performance during Exercise." *Clinical Therapeutics* 13, no. 3 (1991): 373–82.

Siddons, L. "'Cocktail' Shelves Maradona: Drugs Lead to Banishment." *Commercial Appeal,* July 1, 1994, p. D1.

"Studies Hint Garlic Cuts Cholesterol." *The Evansville* (Ind.) *Courier,* 1 October 1993, C16.

Toubro, S., A. Astrup, L. Breum, et al. "The Acute and Chronic Effects of Ephedrine/Caffeine Mixtures on Energy Expenditure and Glucose Metabolism in Humans." *International Journal of Obesity Related Metabolic Disorders* 17, Suppl. 3 (1993): 73–77.

Tyler, V. E. "Should Herbal Remedies Remain in FDA Regulatory Limbo?" *Nutrition Forum* 9, no. 6 (1992): 41–46.

Vanherweghem, J. L., M. Depierreux, C. Tielemans, et al. "Rapidly Progressive Interstitial Renal Fibrosis in Young Women: Association with Slimming Regimen Including Chinese Herbs." *The Lancet* 341, no. 8842 (1993): 387–90.

Note: Much of the information in this chapter is adapted from Kleiner, S. M. "Controversial Practices in Sports." In *Sports Nutrition: A Guide for the Professional Working with Active People.* 2d ed., edited by D. Benardot. Chicago: The American Dietetic Association, 1993.

Chapter 14: Caffeine

Benardot, D., ed. *Sports Nutrition: A Guide for the Professional Working with Active People.* 2d ed. Chicago: The American Dietetic Association, 1993.

Clark, N. "What's Brewing with Caffeine?" *The Physician and Sportsmedicine* 2 (1994): 15–16.

Engels, H-J., and E. M. Haymes. "Effects of Caffeine Ingestion on Metabolic Responses to Prolonged Walking in Sedentary Males." *International Journal of Sport Nutrition* 2 (1992): 386–96.

Graham, T. E., and L. L. Spriet. "Metabolic Catecholamine, and Exercise Performance Responses to Various Doses of Caffeine." *Journal of Applied Physiology* 78, no. 3 (1995): 867–74.

Jackman, M., P. Wendling, D. Friars, et al. "Caffeine Ingestion and High-Intensity Intermittent Exercise." Personal communication with Larry Spriet, University of Guelph, Ontario, Canada.

Massey, L. K., E. A. Bergman, K. J. Wise, et al. "Interactions between Dietary Caffeine and Calcium on Bone Metabolism in Older Women." *Journal of the American College of Nutrition* 13 (1994): 592–96.

McMurtry, J. J., and R. Sherwin. "History, Pharmacology, and Toxiology of Caffeine and Caffeine-Containing Beverages. *Clinical Nutrition* 6 (1987): 249–54.

Mills, J. L., L. B. Homes, J. H. Aarons, et al. "Moderate Caffeine Use and the Risk of Spontaneous Abortion and Intrauterine Growth Retardation. *Journal of the American Medical Association* 269 (1993): 593–97.

VanSoeren, M. H., P. Sathaasviam, L. Spriet, et al. "Caffeine Metabolism and Epinephrine Responses in Users and Nonusers." *Journal of Applied Physiology* 75, no. 2 (1993): 805–12.

Chapter 15: Water

Brouns, F., W. Saris, and H. Schneider. "Rationale for Upper Limits of Electrolyte Replacement during Exercise." *International Journal of Sport Nutrition* 2 (1992): 229–38.

Coyle, E. F. "Fluid and Carbohydrate Replacement during Exercise: How Much and Why?" *Gatorade Sports Science Institute* 7, no. 3 (1994): 50.

Stamford, B. "Muscle Cramps. Untying the Knots." *The Physician and Sportsmedicine* 21 (1993): 115–16.

Chapter 16: Sports Drinks

"Benefits of Fluid Replacement with Carbohydrate during Exericise." *Medicine and Science in Sports and Exercise* 24 (1992): S324–S330.

Coyle, E. F., and S. J. Montain. "Carbohydrate and Fluid Ingestion During Exercise: Are There Trade-Offs?" *Medicine and Science in Sports and Exercise* 24 (1992): 671–78.

Lukaski, H. "Micronutrients: Are Mineral Supplements Necessary in the Athlete's Diet?" Paper presented at the Nutritional Ergogenic Aids Conference sponsored by the Gatorade Sports Institute, November 11–12, 1994, Chicago.

Pacelli, L. C. "Carbohydrate Drinks: Are They Ergogenic?" *The Physician and Sportsmedicine* 18, no. 3 (1990): 50.

Chapter 17: Do You Need to Lose Weight?

Folson, A. R., S. A. Kaye, T. A. Sellers, et al. "Body Fat Distribution and 5-Year Risk of Death in Older Women." *Journal of the American Medical Association* 269, no. 4 (1993): 483–87. Reported by Smith, C. R. "Fat Distribution Linked to Mortality Risk." *The Physician and Sportsmedicine* 21, no. 5 (1993): 40.

Chapter 18: Successful Weight Control

Dattilo, A. M. "Dietary Fat and Its Relationship to Body Weight." *Nutrition Today* 27 (1992): 13–19.

Oscar, L. B., M. M. Brown, and W. C. Miller. "Effect of Dietary Fat on Food Intake, Growth, and Body Composition in Rats." *Growth* 48 (1984): 415–24.

Ravussin, E., S. Lillioja, W. C. Knowler, et al. "Reduced Energy Expenditure as a Risk Factor for Body-Weight Gain." *New England Journal of Medicine* 318 (1988): 467–72.

Tucker, L. A., and M. J. Kano. "Dietary Fat and Body Fat: A Multivariate Study of 205 Adult Females." *American Journal of Clinical Nutrition* 56, no. 4 (1992): 616–22.

Van Zant, R. S. "Influence of Diet and Exercise on Energy Expenditure—A Review." *International Journal of Sport Nutrition* 2 (1992): 1–19.

Chapter 19: Lifestyle Diet Planning

Fadiman, C., ed. *The Little Brown Book of Anecdotes.* Boston: Little, Brown, 1985 (p. 61).

Chapter 20: Sugar and Fat Substitutes

"A Fat Substitute That Lowers Cholesterol." *American Health,* September 1994: 92.

Associated Press. "Fake Fat Tastes the Same but Has Fewer Calories." *The Evansville* (Ind.) *Courier*, 19 April 1994.

Calorie Control Council. "Use of Light Products Growing Fastest among Older Americans." *Calorie Control Commentary* 16, no. 2 (1994): 6.

U.S. Department of Health and Human Services. Public Health Service. *The Surgeon General's Report on Nutrition and Health,* #88/50210, 1988, 277.

Chapter 21: The Role of Exercise in Fat Loss

Anderson, O. "Burn, Baby, Burn." *Runner's World,* May 1995, 38.

Gillette, C. A., R. C. Bullough, and C. L. Melby. "Postexercise Energy Expenditure in Response to Acute Aerobic or Resistive Exercise." *International Journal of Sport Nutrition* 4 (1994): 347–60.

Svendsen, O. L., C. Hassager, and C. Christiansen. "Effect of an Energy-Restrictive Diet, with or without Exercise, on Lean Tissue Mass, Resting Metabolic Rate, Cardiovascular Risk Factors, and Bone in Overweight Postmenopausal Women." *American Journal of Medicine* 95, no. 2 (1993): 131–40.

Chapter 22: If You Want to Maintain or Gain Weight

Harberson, D. A. "Weight Gain and Body Composition of Weightlifters: Effect of High-Calorie Supplementation vs Anabolic Steroids." In *Muscle Development: Nutritional Alternatives to Anabolic Steroids,* edited by W. E. Garrett, Jr. and T. E. Malone. Columbus, OH: Ross Laboratories, 1988.

Haus, G., S. L. Hoerr, B. Mavis, and J. Robison. "Key Modifiable Factors in Weight Maintenance: Fat Intake, Exercise, and Weight Cycling." *Journal of the American Dietetic Association* 94, no. 4 (1994): 409–13.

Chapter 23: High-Performance Vegetarian Nutrition

Althoff, S. "Meatless Muscle: Vegetarian Bodybuilders Bulk Up Just Fine without the Beef." *Vegetarian Times* 200 (1994): 69–73.

Chang-Claude, J., and R. Frentzel-Beyme. "Dietary and Lifestyle Determinants of Mortality among German Vegetarians." *International Journal of Epidemiology* 22, no. 2 (1993): 228–36.

DeSilver, D., V. Moran, and C. Wiley. "Vegetarians Under the Microscope: Medical Research 1974–1990." *Vegetarian Times* 160 (1990): 50–60.

Geil, P. B., and J. W. Anderson. "Nutrition and Health Implications of Dry Beans: A Review." *Journal of the American College of Nutrition* 13 (1994): 549–58.

Gorman, M. A., and C. Bowman. "Position of the American Dietetic Association: Health Implications of Dietary Fiber." *Journal of the American Dietetic Association* 93 (1993): 1446–47.

Hanninen, O., M. Nenonen, W. H. Ling, et al. "Effects of eating an uncooked vegetable diet for one week." *Appetite* 19, no. 3 (1992): 243–54.

Havala, S. "Vegetarian Diets—Clearing the Air." *The Western Journal of Medicine* 160, no. 5 (1994): 483–84.

Kleiner, S. "Veg Pledge." *Female Bodybuilding,* July 1993, 16–18.

Levine, A. S., J. R. Tallman, M. K. Grace, S. A. Parker, C. J. Billington, and M. D. Levitt. "Effect of Breakfast Cereals on Short-Term Food Intake." *American Journal of Clinical Nutrition* 50 (1989): 1303–07.

Liebman, B. "Fear of Bloating: Beans Needn't Be Bland or Embarrassing." *Nutrition Action Newsletter* (1983): 12–14.

Mead, N. "Special Report: 6500 Chinese Can't Be Wrong." *Vegetarian Times* 158 (1990): 15–17.

Raben, A., B. Kiens, E. A. Richter, et al. "Serum Sex Hormones and Endurance Performance after a Lacto-Ovo Vegetarian Diet and a Mixed Diet." *Medicine and Science in Sports and Exercise* 24, no. 11 (1992): 1290–97.

Rivers, J. M., and K. K. Collins. *Planning Meals That Lower Cancer Risk: A Reference Guide.* Washington, DC: American Institute for Cancer Research. 1984.

Scharffenberg, J. "Living a Longer, Healthier, and Happier Life." *Vibrant Life* 8, no. 3 (1992): 16–18.

Weaver, C. M., and K. L. Plawecki. "Dietary Calcium: Adequacy of a Vegetarian Diet." *American Journal of Clinical Nutrition* 59 (1994): 1238–41.

White, R., and E. Frank. "Health Effects and Prevalence of Vegetarianism." *The Western Journal of Medicine* 160, no. 5 (1994): 465–71.

Chapter 24: Nutrition during Pregnancy

Jacobson, M. F., L. Y. Lefferts, and A. W. Garland. *Safe Food: Eating Wisely in a Risky World.* Los Angeles: Center for Science in the Public Interest and Living Planet Press, 1991.

Kleiner, S. M., and K. R. Friedman-Kester. "Special Nutritional Needs through the Life Cycle." In *Clinical Preventive Medicine,* edited by R. S. Matzen and R. S. Lang. St. Louis: Mosby-Year Book, Inc., 1993.

Mills, J. L., B. I. Graubard, E. E. Harley, G. G. Rhoads, and H. W. Berendes. "Maternal Alcohol Consumption and Birth Weight: How Much Drinking During Pregnancy Is Safe?" *Journal of the American Medical Association* 252 (1984): 1875–79.

MRC Vitamin Study Research Group. "Prevention of Neural Tube Defects: Results of the Medical Research Council Vitamin Study." *Lancet* 338 (1991): 131–37.

National Research Council. *Recommended Dietary Allowances,* 10th ed. Washington, DC: National Academy Press, 1989.

U. S. Department of Health and Human Services. Public Health Service. *The Surgeon General's Report on Nutrition and Health.* Publication No. 88-50210. Washington, DC: GPO, 1988.

Chapter 25: High Performance through the Ages

Associated Press. "Pumping Iron Builds Up Bones in Older Women, Study Finds." *The Evansville* (Ind.) *Courier,* 28 December 1994, A7

Bland, J. S. "How Young Are You? Good Habits, Nutrition and Antioxidants Can Slow Down Biological Aging." *Health News & Review* 3, no. 2 (1993): A.

"Body Building for the Nineties." Interview with William Evans, Department of Agriculture's Human Nutrition Research Center on Aging. *Nutrition Action Health Letter* 19, no. 5 (1992): 1–3.

Council on Scientific Affairs, American Medical Association. "Diet and Cancer: Where Do Matters Stand?" *Archives of Internal Medicine* 153 (1993): 50–56.

"Daily Vitamins Boost Immunity." *Harvard Health Letter,* May 1993, 4–5.

Fiatarone, M. A., E. C. Marks, N. D. Ryan, C. N. Meredith, L. A. Lipsitz, and W. J. Evans. "High-Intensity Strength Training in Nonagenarians." *Journal of the American Medical Association* 263 (1990): 3029–34.

"For Your Heart's Sake, More B Vitamins." *Tufts University Diet & Nutrition Letter* 11, no. 12 (1994): 1–2.

Friedlander, A. L., and H. K. Genant. "Positive Response of the Skeleton to Exercise Intervention in Young Women." *Journal of Bone Mineral Research* 7, suppl. 1 (1992): 5321. Reported by Mannings, F. "Building Bone Beyond the Teen Years." *The Physician and Sportsmedicine* 21, no. 1 (1993): 15–16.

Gersten, A. "Effect of Exercise on Muscle Function Decline with Aging." *The Western Journal of Medicine* 154, no. 5 (1991): 579–82.

Liebman, B. "Designer Foods." *Nutrition Action Newsletter* 19, no. 4 (1992): 1–4.

McBean, L. D., T. Forgac, and S. C. Finn. "Osteoporosis: Visions for Care and Prevention—A Conference Report." *Journal of the American Dietetic Association* 94, no. 6 (1994): 668–71.

Rosenberg, I. H. "Nutritional Needs of the Elderly." In *Nutrition Research: Future Directions and Applications,* edited by J. E. Fielding and H. I. Frier. New York: Raven Press, 1991.

Toufexis, A. "The New Scoop on Vitamins." *Time,* 6 April 1992, 54–59.

Webb, A. R., L. Kline, and M. F. Holick. "Influence of Season and Latitude on the Cutaneous Synthesis of Vitamin D_3: Exposure to Winter Sunlight in Boston and Edmonton Will Not Promote Vitamin D_3 Synthesis in Human Skin." *Journal of Clinical Endocrinology and Metabolism* 61 (1988): 373–78.

Appendix D: Medication and Nutrition Guide

Powers, D. E., and A. O. Moore. *Food Medication Interactions.* A Pocketbook. 5th ed. Phoenix: Food-Medication Interactions, 1986.

Appendix F: Food Additives

"Food Preservative May Rev Up Anti-Cancer Gene." *The Evansville* (Ind.) *Courier,* 13 September 1994, A16.

Jacobson, M. *Safe Food.* Venice, CA: Center for Science in the Public Interest and Living Planet Press, 1991.

Index